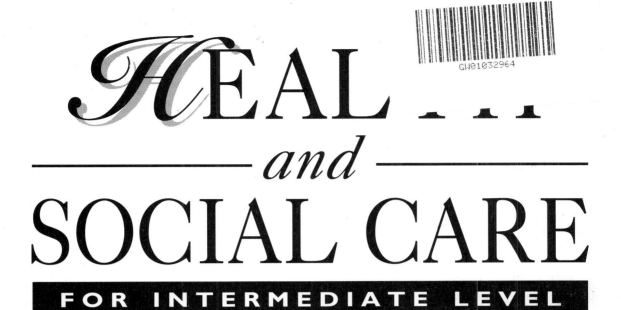

HEALTH
and
SOCIAL CARE
FOR INTERMEDIATE LEVEL

Edited by

SUE BENSON

Hodder & Stoughton

A MEMBER OF THE HODDER HEADLINE GROUP

ACKNOWLEDGEMENTS

The authors would like to thank their families and friends for their support and encouragement.

For the reproduction of copyright material, the publishers would like to thank the following: the Health Education Authority for the inclusion of nutritional guidelines in Chapter 1, table 1.1 and fig 1.5; Alex Huber/Impact, fig 1.3; Jenny Matthews/Save the Children, fig 1.4; C. Stacher/Photofusion, fig 1.7; Martin Black/Impact, fig 1.13; Sarah Wild/Photofusion, fig 2.2; Sally & Richard Greenhill, figs 2.3, 2.8, 2.9, 7.6, 8.1; Bruce Stephens/Impact, fig 2.5; Joanne O'Brien/Format, fig 2.6; Brenda Prince/Format, figs 2.10, 4.4; Judy Harrison/Format, 2.12; Sam Tanner/Photofusion, figs 3.1, 4.8, 8.2; Age Concern, fig 3.2; Department of Health, figs 3.5, 3.7, 3.8, 7.2, 7.4 (all crown copyright); John Cole/Impact, fig 3.9; Maggie Murray/Format, fig 4.2; Crispin Hughes/Photofusion, fig 4.5; Peter Arkell/Impact, figs 6.2, 8.3; SCOPE, fig 6.4; Paula Solloway/Format, fig 6.6; Frank Watson/Photofusion, fig 6.7; Ralph Erle/Impact, fig 6.10; Vale Royal Careline, The Sheltered Housing Service, Northwich, fig 6.12; Stannah Stairlifts Ltd, fig 6.13; Ortho-Kinetics (UK) Ltd, fig 6.14; The Special Collection, fig 6.15; Mo Wilson/Format, fig 8.4.

Every effort has been made to trace the copyright holders of material reproduced in this book. Any rights omitted from the acknowledgements here or in the text will be added for subsequent printings following notice to the publisher.

A catalogue record for this title is available from the British Library

ISBN 0 340 620579

First published 1996
Impression number 10 9 8 7 6 5 4 3 2 1
Year   2000 1999 1998 1997 1996

Typeset by Wearset, Boldon, Tyne and Wear.
Printed in Great Britain for Hodder & Stoughton Educational, a division of Hodder Headline Plc, 338 Euston Road, London NW1 3BH by the Bath Press, Avon.

Joanne Hills.

CONTENTS

AUTHOR DETAILS

Liz Day
Chapter 1, Promoting health and well-being, and Chapter 2, Influences on health and well-being
Senior lecturer, Health Studies, Croydon College

Jill Cowley
Chapter 1, Promoting health and well-being
Senior practice nurse, Lincolnshire

Esther Parker
Chapter 2, Influences on health and well-being
Programme coordinator, Child Health, Thames Valley University

Brenda Hooper
Chapter 3, Health and Social Care Services
Consultant and trainer in residential care

Sebastian Randall
Chapter 4, Communication and interpersonal relationships, and Chapter 2, Influences on health and well-being
Psychotherapist and lecturer in counselling, Essex

Jo Newman
Chapter 5, Application of science in health and social care
Lecturer, Thomas Danby College, Leeds

Alan Skelt
Chapter 6, Meeting the needs of individuals in different care settings
Social worker, Cheshire

Tessa Perrin
Chapter 7, Creative activities in care settings
Senior practitioner occupational therapist and researcher, Bradford Dementia Group

Linda Nazarko
Chapter 8, Practical caring skills
Matron of a nursing home, Surrey

INTRODUCTION

WHAT IS A GNVQ?

A General National Vocational Qualification is a broad based qualification which tests understanding of a vocational area – in your case, health and social care.

GNVQs are currently available at three levels:

- Foundation
- Intermediate
- Advanced.

You may have already completed a Foundation level course before starting Intermediate, or you may be starting your first GNVQ course. In either case, you will have several options at the end of the course. You can either continue with your GNVQ studies, by taking the Advanced level course, or you can seek work in the health and care field.

HOW IS THE INTERMEDIATE GNVQ STRUCTURED?

Units

The intermediate qualification is split into six vocational units and three core skills units. Four of the vocational units are mandatory, and must be done by everyone. They are:

- Promoting health and well-being
- Influences on health and well-being
- Health and social care services
- Communication and interpersonal relationships in health and social care.

These units relate to the first four chapters of the book.

You must then take two option units, chosen from a list of four. The option units depend on which awarding body your school or college is with. This book covers the four option units offered by BTEC (Business and Technology Education Council), and it is likely that you will cover two of these options from this book. They are:

- Application of science in health and social care
- Meeting the needs of individuals in different care settings
- Creative activities in care settings
- Practical caring skills.

Elements

Each unit is broken down into elements. For example, unit 1, 'Promoting health and well-being', has three elements:

1.1   Investigate personal health

1.2 Present advice on health and well-being to others

1.3 Reduce risk of injury and deal with emergencies

These are broad headings which explain what the overall unit is about. The elements will help you understand what you are expected to do, understand, or achieve. Each chapter of the book covers all the elements of the unit, in the order in which they are listed in the syllabus.

Performance criteria

Each element is then broken down into smaller parts, called performance criteria. For example, in element 1.1, 'Investigate personal health' there are 6 performance criteria:

1 Explain the importance of a *balanced* lifestyle
2 Explain risks and benefits associated with *aspects of lifestyle*
3 Identify how the body uses each dietary *component*
4 Describe a *healthy diet* for an *individual*
5 Describe the *effects* of use of substances on health and well-being
6 Explain good practice in maintaining *hygiene*

These are the specific things you will be expected to do, understand or achieve in each element.

Range

You will see that some words within the performance criteria are highlighted in bold. These key words and phrases are explained in greater detail under the heading 'Range'. For instance, you will find a list of what kinds of *aspects of lifestyle* or what sort of *individual* you are expected to cover:

- *Aspects of lifestyle* exercise, diet (adequate, balanced), sufficient rest, smoking, alcohol, sexual behaviour including celibacy.
- *Individual* active, sedentary, child, elderly person, pregnant woman.

WHAT MUST I DO TO PASS AN INTERMEDIATE GNVQ?

Portfolio of evidence

You must gather evidence to show that you can do, understand or achieve the performance criteria within each element, within each unit. In order to do this, you will need to carry out activities or tasks, and keep the results together in a portfolio of evidence.

For your final assessment, you will not need to present every single piece of evidence collected. You will however need to have assignments covering each evidence indicator which has been written. There is currently one for each element, and so you will need some evidence for each element.

Examples of evidence you will need to collect and keep are:

- written reports
- diaries
- statistics that you have collected
- video or audio cassettes
- presentations
- photographs
- letters and memos
- assessment of previous achievements and qualifications
- written statements or testimonials (especially if you are able to carry out a work placement)

- evidence from work experience or part-time employment

You will need to organise your own portfolio of evidence right from the start. It will help if you have a large folder, and some subject dividers. You will need to have sections for the following:

- one section for each mandatory unit (4)
- one section for each optional unit (2)
- one section for each core skill (3)

That is a total of nine main sections. Within the main sections, you should have subsections for each element of the unit – usually three, sometimes four:

- one section for any additional forms or material needed by your school, college or awarding body
- a contents list – at the beginning!

Where the same evidence can be used in more than one place (e.g. for a vocational element *and* a core skill element), you should put it in one place only. You can then refer back to it where it would appear the second time (cross reference).

End test

You will also need to pass an end test made up of multiple choice questions. There is one test for each of the four mandatory units: they each last for one hour and have about 30–40 questions. Tests are held several times a year, and you can take a particular unit test more than once – indeed, as often as you need to. You need to get 70% of the multiple choice questions right to pass, but with practice you should get through, even if not the first time round.

HOW DO I IMPROVE MY GRADES?

Grades of merit and distinction are awarded on the basis of your portfolio of evidence only – the end test at present is simply pass or fail. If one third of your portfolio meets the requirement for a higher grade, then you can be awarded a merit or distinction. There are two main themes on which your work will be assessed – *Process* (how you do your work) and *Outcomes* (what the results are). There are three themes under the Process heading:

- Planning
- Information seeking and information handling
- Evaluation

There is one theme under the Outcomes heading:

- Quality of outcomes

What grade you are awarded will depend on how you carried out your work within these grading themes. The list below shows what exactly is involved for each theme. The more you carry out on your own, changing a plan where necessary or asking questions about how successful your work was, the more likely you are to achieve a higher grade.

Planning

- drawing up plans of action
- monitoring courses of action

Points to consider: how much advice do you need to draw up your action plan? What will you do if it goes wrong?

Information seeking and information handling

- identifying and using sources to obtain information
- establishing the validity of information

Points to consider: can you work out for yourself where to find out what you need to know? How will you check the information that you discover — is there somewhere else where you can check your facts?

Evaluation

- evaluating outcomes and alternatives
- justifying particular approaches to tasks or activities

Points to consider: was the outcome what you expected, or not? Do you know why? Can you explain why you carried out your assignment in the way that you did?

Quality of outcomes

- synthesis (combining different pieces of information)
- command of 'language'

Points to consider: can you put all your results together and draw a conclusion? How well can you present your findings to other people, and does your report use the terms and phrases used by those working in health and social care?

CORE SKILLS

We mentioned before that as well as taking four mandatory and two optional units, you must collect evidence for three core skills units. These are:

- Communication
- Application of number
- Information technology.

With one mandatory unit and a core skill devoted to communication, you will see that a great deal of emphasis is placed on this issue within health and social care. It is a tremendously important skill to gain if you are eventually going to work with people who need support and care.

All three skills however are a key part of your course. The evidence you collect to show that you have covered the elements required, should come from the assignments you carry out for the mandatory and optional units: i.e. you need to practise the core skills within the context of health and social care.

The elements for each core skill unit are as follows:

Communication

- take part in discussions
- produce written material
- use images
- read and respond to written materials

Application of number

- collect and record data
- tackle problems
- interpret and present data

Information technology

- prepare information
- process information
- present information
- evaluate the use of information technology

You should use these skills where possible in your activities, tasks and assignments, and keep a record of when you do so.

1

PROMOTING HEALTH AND WELL-BEING

AIMS AND OBJECTIVES

The aim of this chapter is to consider ways in which health can be improved by both health promotion and harm reduction strategies.

By the end of this chapter you will be able to:

- explain the importance of a balanced lifestyle

- explain the risks and the benefits associated with the choices we make

- present advice on health and well-being to others

- know how to reduce the risk of injury and deal with emergencies

---

Investigating personal health

This section will look at the ways in which individuals, as part of their everyday lives, undertake particular courses of action which are aimed at maintaining their personal health. Some of the actions taken may result in an element of risk, such as cycling and swimming, but on the whole, people weigh up the risks and benefits before embarking on such activities.

Considering the personal implications of action may take the form of thinking things through, or talking them over with others. In thinking and talking about our actions in this way, we are accepting responsibility for

them. These pages will discuss this process and the way in which you may help others to make informed choices, even if the choice is not necessarily what you consider to be the 'right' choice. It will also help you to assess the health and well-being of others, plan ways in which health may be improved, present advice and also assess the effect of that advice. This element does not look at the way our lifestyles or the choices which we appear to make freely, are influenced by external pressures and policies beyond our control. This will be discussed in Chapter 2.

PERSONAL RESPONSIBILITY

A healthy lifestyle is important if we want to pursue our aims and ambitions in life. People attempt to look after their own health in many different ways. These need to be respected and taken into account when you are giving advice to others. The following activity will enable you to reflect on ways in which you try to live a healthy life and enhance your well-being.

Activity 1

Write down all the different things you do to promote your own health. When you have done this, ask family members of different age groups what measures they take to protect or maintain their health.

COMMENT

Compare your list with other people's lists and also compare them with the list below, which is by no means conclusive and in no particular order.

Health promoting activities may include:

- eating a balanced diet
- restricting alcohol consumption
- eating a moderate amount of sweet food
- not taking illegal drugs
- obtaining advice on over-the-counter medication
- seeking medical advice when unwell, if necessary
- seeking specific advice for particular situations, such as during pregnancy, before travelling abroad, etc.
- maintaining personal hygiene standards, including dental care

- skin care, such as sun block creams, or keeping covered in very hot weather
- wearing clothing and footwear appropriate to the weather (with an eye on fashion as well perhaps)
- making sure you have enough sleep
- having immunisations
- taking regular exercise
- making time to relax and enjoy yourself
- pursuing sport and/or leisure activities
- talking over problems with friends, family and counsellors
- forming and maintaining relationships (and breaking them if they are hurtful, destructive or incompatible)
- protecting yourself or your partner against unwanted pregnancy or sexually transmitted diseases
- learning first aid
- taking care of pets
- driving carefully with seat belts worn
- taking up new challenges
- reading
- learning new skills
- practising your spiritual and cultural beliefs
- keeping in touch with friends
- being aware of Health and Safety practices at work
- weighing up the risks and benefits before taking action

These are just some of the possibilities for promoting your own health. No doubt you will have found many more examples from the people you interviewed. You may have noticed some differences between people depending on their age, gender and other personal factors, but there are many similarities in the ways in which we take care of ourselves.

You will see quite clearly that these possible answers cover more than just taking care of the body or physical health. They include taking care of social relationships, mental health, spiritual well-being, and the environment. We shall now look at the first few examples of self health promotion on the list. These relate to physical health, and include diet, fluid intake and alcohol consumption.

A BALANCED DIET

People often talk about a 'diet' as if it is something special which we do in order to lose weight or control a condition such as diabetes (sugar intolerance). A diet is a general term to cover any foods which we eat, including food to help us lose weight or control a medical condition. People also talk about a 'healthy diet' and it is often assumed that everyone is talking about the same thing – but they may not be.

Activity 2

Ask a retired person, a working person who participates in an active sport and a parent (of either sex) what they think are the basic nutritional requirements which they and their family need to be healthy. In other words, find out what they think is a 'healthy' diet. Write down their answers and compare with the guidelines below.

COMMENT

Remember that these are only guidelines. *We are individuals of different ages, with different tastes, cultures, preferences, religions, physical activities and perhaps have physical conditions which require advice and guidance from a qualified dietician, doctor, nurse or health adviser.*

We also have different levels of income which will influence what we can afford to eat and how we prepare food. We live in different areas which affect the availability of foods.

We all need a selection of foods from four main food groups:

1 **Bread, cereals, potatoes** This group includes breakfast cereals, pitta bread, chapati, cracker biscuits, rice, pasta, noodles, plantain, green banana, sweet potatoes. These foods give us energy for everyday activities and contain essential vitamins (to be discussed later). Whether people need more or less of this food group depends on the nature of their work and their leisure activities. As a general rule everyone should have food from this group on a daily basis.

2 **Vegetable and fruit** Different foods include salads, fruit (fresh, tinned and frozen), cooked fruit, fruit juices, cooked and raw vegetables, vegetable soups. These are a rich source of minerals and vitamins as well as energy and fibre: some foods from this group should be eaten daily.

3 **Milk and dairy** This group consists of milk, yoghurt, fromage frais, cottage cheese, and cheese. These and the next food group are important for body maintenance, growth and repair.

4 **Meat and alternatives** This includes chicken, pork, ham, lamb, liver, kidney, fish, eggs, pulses, lentils or dhal, baked beans, nuts or nut products like peanut butter.

People also need fats such as butter, margarine, low-fat spreads, cooking oil, lard, dripping, ghee or mayonnaise, but we are recommended by government reports to cut down on these products. Eating these foods too often may lead to us being overweight (obese) and to increasing our risk of developing coronary heart disease (see Table 1.1 below).

You will see that the food groups above do not include many of the things which are eaten daily as snacks or treats. Our consumption of fatty or sugary foods should be limited. This means that we have to take a different approach when we want a quick snack. Instead of opening a packet of crisps or a chocolate bar, we need to get into the habit of eating a piece of fruit, or a pitta bread with a nutritious filling (something from the food groups above). Temptation is all around us though – supermarkets which have chocolate eggs and packs of sweets at the check-out tills. As we wait patiently to be served, somehow sweets seem to find their way into our shopping trolley!

It is well known that eating too much sugary food can cause us to be overweight, which may in turn lead to lack of exercise, high blood pressure, diabetes, bad teeth and other health problems. So why, when we know the risks, do we choose to eat chocolate and sweets?

Activity 3

 Jot down some benefits of buying and eating sweets.

COMMENT

 You may have noted that sweets:

- are a very easily accessible food source (a quick answer to hunger)

- can be shared with others: the offering of sweets may be a sign of friendship and love

- may be given to someone as a gift on birthdays and other occasions

- are a fairly cheap yet luxury item

- taste good

It would be unreasonable to suggest that sweets are banished from our diet. This is why it was suggested in Activity 1 that eating a moderate amount of sweet food, as part of our approach to adopting a healthy lifestyle, was probably better than saying sweets should be banned. This means that we need to consider carefully our overall consumption of different foods, and the benefits and risks involved in indulging ourselves. Only then can we decide whether or not the risks

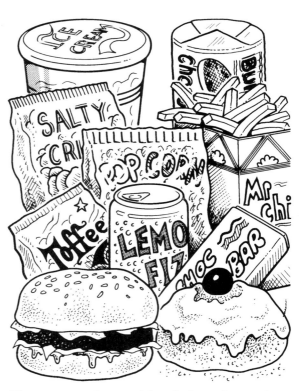

Figure 1.1   *Sweet and fatty foods may be tasty, but too much is bad for our health*

Table 1.1 Changing what you eat

What's in a measure?	Daily measures	What counts as a measure?
Bread, cereal and potato group	5–11 include some wholegrain products daily	• 3 tbs breakfast cereal • slice of bread/toast • ½ bread bun/roll • small pitta bread/chapati • 3 crackers • egg-sized potato • rice/pasta/noodles (2 tbs) • plantain, green banana or sweet potatoes (2 tbs)
Vegetable and fruit group	5–9 include a mixture of vegetables and fruits daily	• vegetables (2 tbs) • small salad • piece of fresh fruit e.g. an apple or an orange • stewed/tinned fruit (2 tbs) • small (100 ml) fruit juice
Milk and dairy group	2–3 choose lower fat types	• 200 ml/⅓ pint milk • small pot yoghurt, cottage cheese or fromage frais • 1½ oz/40 g cheese (small matchbox-sized)
Meat and alternatives group	2–3 choose lower fat types	• 2–3 oz/50–70 g beef, pork, ham, lamb, liver, kidney/chicken or oily fish • 4–5 oz/100–150 g white fish (not fried in batter) • 2 eggs (up to 6 per week) • 200 g or 3 tbs baked beans, pulses, lentils or dhal • 1½ oz/40 g cheese (small matchbox-sized) • 60 g or 2 tbs nuts or nut products (e.g. peanut butter)
Fats	0–3 measures daily	• 1 tsp butter/margarine • 2 tsp low-fat spread • 1 tsp cooking oil, lard, dripping or ghee • 1 tsp mayonnaise or oily salad dressing
Fatty and sugary foods	limit to 1 daily	sugar (e.g. in drinks), fatty bacon, sausages, luncheon meat, pork pie, sausage roll, crisps, biscuits, rich sauces, fatty gravies, cream, creamy cheese, doughnut, Danish pastry, pie, cake, ice-cream, chocolate

Reproduced with permission from the Health Education Authority.

outweigh the benefits. You might like to consider the advantages and disadvantages of eating sweets and sweet foods. Some of these are included in the comments under Activity 7 later in this chapter.

To maintain a balanced and healthy diet, we need to select some foods from each of the four groups each day, but the amounts or numbers of measures depend upon whether we are female or male, our age, weight, activity levels and overall health. A general guide can be found in Table 1.1 on page 9 but more specific guidance can be obtained from the dietician, general practitioner, nurse or health visitor at the local health centre.

Vitamins

You may be wondering where vitamins fit in, and whether we should take vitamin tablets as a general rule. Generally speaking, if you eat foods from each of the food groups every day, you are healthy and have no special requirements because of pregnancy for example, or a specific health problem, you should not need to take extra vitamins, because the vitamins you need are in the foods you eat. Have a look at the list below:

- **Vitamin A** – keeps skin and the linings of the mouth, throat, stomach and other organs healthy and helps us to see colours and see at night. It is found in liver, milk and milk products, butter, eggs, carrots and dark green leafy vegetables.
- **Vitamin B** – (there are several vitamins in the Vitamin B group) is necessary for healthy blood cells, nervous system and the digestion of proteins. It is found in milk, meat, cereals, eggs, meat and meat products, cheese, fish, liver, potatoes, bread, and egg.
- **Vitamin C** – helps to keep muscles and tendons strong and healthy and enables us to produce certain hormones in the body.

It is present in potatoes, fruits and fruit juices, citrus fruits and green vegetables.
- **Vitamin D** – helps our bones and teeth to grow strong and healthy, it helps repair broken bones and is also responsible for our absorption of calcium. Foods containing Vitamin D include dairy produce and oily fish.
- **Vitamin E** – is necessary for healthy cell growth in our body and is found in vegetable oils, cereals, eggs and dark green leafy vegetables.
- **Vitamin K** – helps our blood to clot when we cut ourselves and also helps us to transform food we eat into energy. Vitamin K is found in vegetables such as sprouts, cabbage, cauliflower and spinach.

Minerals

As well as vitamins, we need certain minerals. Iron and calcium are the most commonly known. Minerals are important for health and are found in different foods from the four food groups. It is beyond the scope of this chapter to go into a great deal of detail; you should refer to books written specifically about diet and by dieticians. Find out from the receptionist of a general practice where the local dietician works, and discuss with him or her the kind of services on offer and the sorts of problems with which they are able to help.

ALCOHOL, TOBACCO AND HEALTH

You may have noticed that alcohol does not appear in any of the food groups. Alcohol contains calories which contribute a great deal to our weight without contributing to our nutrition. In its Health of the Nation targets, the government is aiming to encour-

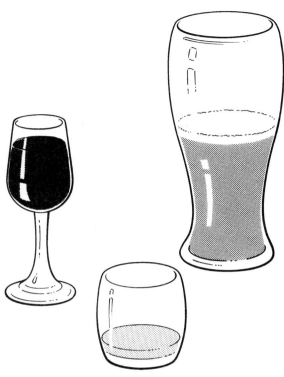

Figure 1.2   *A unit of alcohol: half a pint of beer, a small glass of wine, a measure of spirits*

age us to reduce our regular intake of alcohol. The Sensible Drinking Report published in December 1995 recommends that to avoid significant health problems, men should drink no more than 3–4 units of alcohol per day, whereas women should not drink over 2–3 units of alcohol per day.

Alcohol is not a necessary part of a diet, and may contribute unwanted calories and thus weight gain. It is said to be one of the most socially acceptable 'drugs' on the market. It affects the way in which we act and think, and so should be treated with caution. Such is the effect of alcohol on our judgement and our thinking, that it is illegal to drink more than a small amount of alcohol before driving, and it is unwise to drink before many other activities such as swimming. Alcohol may also affect our behaviour,

perhaps making us less inhibited and more aggressive. It can also become addictive if consumed regularly.

However, alcohol does have some benefits:

1 It is pleasant to drink on social occasions, such as weddings and parties.

2 It may be shared with others, or given as a gift (a bottle of wine is often given as a Christmas present).

3 People often feel more relaxed after a drink, and are less shy in social situations.

Clearly, drinking alcohol in some circumstances can be quite pleasant.

Cigarette smoking is often associated with alcohol. Tobacco has had a remarkable history: it has been hailed as 'a good thing' on the one hand, and a real health risk on the other. It was provided free to the troops during the last world wars. However as more information has become available about the effects of smoking tobacco, research has made clear that there is no such thing as a safe cigarette.

Activity 4

Have a look at the sporting activities such as cricket, snooker and motor racing on the television. Count how many times the names of various brands of cigarettes appear, and how many sporting activities are sponsored by tobacco companies. At the same time, look out for alcohol advertising in sport.

COMMENT

You may have been surprised at the amount of advertising and sponsorship of sport by tobacco companies and breweries. The link between sport, alcohol and tobacco is financial, as drinking and smoking do not improve our performance at sport

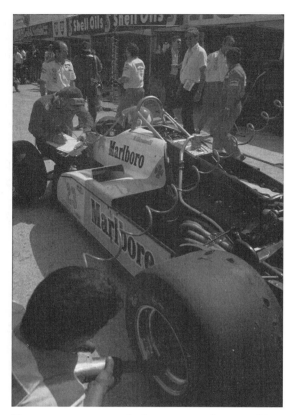

Figure 1.3   *Formula One racing is dominated by tobacco sponsorship*

(although it may make us think we are better than we really are!).

Tobacco advertising on television was banned several years ago. However, you will probably have noticed that sports television programmes often show the background advertising. We do not really know the effects of advertising tobacco and alcohol on people's behaviour, but we can assume that advertisers would not waste their money if it was not effective. What we do know is that people continue to drink alcohol (quite heavily in some instances) and to smoke, despite the evidence that both can seriously affect health.

Activity 5

Ask people you know who either drink, smoke, or do both, what their main reasons are for smoking tobacco and drinking alcohol.

COMMENT

Sometimes people smoke because their friends do, and they want to be part of the group. Young people may smoke because they feel it makes them look more adult. Other people may start smoking as a result of stress, as it may appear to relieve stress. Some young women looking after small children, and who are unable to work because of a lack of childcare facilities say they smoke because it is the only little pleasure they can afford.

People give similar kinds of explanations for their alcohol consumptions. Because it is more socially acceptable these days to drink, rather than smoke, some people's alcohol consumption may gradually increase.

Summary

It is clear that if you have a 'balanced' diet (i.e. a diet which includes foods from each of the food groups), you will have the vitamins you need to keep you healthy. It is important to emphasise that, alongside a balanced diet, we need *at least* six to eight cups of fluid daily, preferably plain water. Keeping healthy is essential as it enables you to enjoy life at every stage, whether at play, work or leisure time.

RECREATION, SPORT, RELAXATION AND LEISURE

You will have noticed that the list of ways of maintaining health discussed in Activity 1 included taking regular exercise, making time for yourself to relax and enjoy yourself, and pursuing sport and/or leisure activities. As well as a balanced diet, it is important to ensure that we have a balanced lifestyle, which includes recreation, sport, relaxation and leisure.

There are five main reasons why leisure and recreation have become more regular features in our daily lives than in the past.

1 The working day has become shorter due to changes in employment legislation and increases in technology.
2 People are now not only living longer because of better housing, food, environmental health measures and a good health service, but they are also in better health when they retire and can expect many years of leisure.
3 There have also been major changes in facilities available for work in the house (e.g. washing machines, tumble dryers, fridges and freezers, microwaves and central heating). This means that household chores and food preparation do not take up so much time or physical effort, although, even in this 'liberated' age, there is still evidence to show that the majority of women who work full-time also do most of the housework. However, without enough physical effort, our muscles tend to get smaller and our bones lighter, making us more vulnerable to ill-health.
4 Clothes were once made in the home, but are now mass produced and available outside the home. Now dress-making and knitting tend to be hobbies rather than central features of domestic chores. People therefore have more free time for leisure activities.
5 Leisure activities such as watching television, reading, listening to music, undertaking home study courses, are more widely available to many people.

These changes not only make recreation and leisure activities in and outside the home a possibility for many people at all stages in their life, they are also essential for a healthy body and mind.

Activity 6

Pause for a moment and think about the different leisure, sports and recreational activities you participate in now, and ones which you would like to do so in the future.

What do you enjoy about the ones you do now and why?

What prevents you from doing activities you would like to do?

Find three people from the same sex as yourself, and three people from the opposite sex. Ask these questions, and compare their answers. Try to obtain the views of people with different abilities and disabilities.

COMMENT

Did you find that you and other people are able to enjoy some leisure activities more easily than others? Talking to friends face to face, in groups, at work, on the phone, or in the pub or club may be fairly easy. Other activities which take some effort, such as going out to have a swim or a walk, may be more difficult e.g. in bad weather, or where the individual has a disability and the environment is not suitably accessible (thereby creating barriers for people with limited mobility). We usually have good intentions and mean to undertake some physical activity but are sometimes put off by certain obstacles.

Advice

It is very easy to give 'good' advice to people about their lifestyle, but when we examine our own lifestyles, we sometimes realise that it is not so easy to put it into practice. There is much we would like to do if only we had the time, the money or the motivation (or perhaps all three).

When offering advice to people, it is also important to value and recognise what they are already doing. It is important to build on what they like doing rather than making a suggestion which does not fit in with their lifestyle, or which is unrealistic.

Leisure activities

You may have found that there was a difference between females and males or between people in different age groups. Some prefer sports such as tennis, golf, swimming, badminton, table tennis, squash and weight training, while others prefer bowls, adult education, gardening, walking, knitting and other crafts, writing and painting. Some of these leisure activities involve co-operation and teamwork, while others can be pursued alone. Whatever the activity, it will contribute to physical health and it is well known that energetic activity releases chemicals in the brain which make us feel better.

Whatever way people prefer to use their leisure time, it is important that they have interests and friends away from the workplace. Work does take up a great deal of time, energy and interest for some people, but it may not be a very permanent situation in a changing economic climate.

At different stages in the lifespan, we are involved in different types of activities.

When you were very young, you and your friends were probably provided with play materials to suit your developmental age. Your parents, teachers and main carers would have enabled you to investigate your environment in a safe manner, take acceptable risks but be protected from dangers. You probably remember walking along walls and balancing carefully so as not to fall off. You may have enjoyed playing games with other children such as football or skipping, as well as undertaking individual pursuits such as reading, painting and drawing. You may remember family games undertaken indoors and you may also remember being taken out to swimming pools, leisure centres and for holidays.

All of these activities stretch the mind and the body and contribute to your learning and physical, mental and social development. These activities may have formed the foundation for your ideas on health and your attitude towards leisure activities now. You may now have work responsibilities which leave little time for recreation and leisure activities. You may walk or cycle where possible, and perhaps leave the car far enough away from work to provide a reasonable amount of exercise a day.

There are many leisure centres and fitness suites now which some people use and enjoy for solitary sport like swimming and weight training, or they may continue to participate in team games which they enjoyed at school (e.g. badminton, football, netball and table tennis). Solitary activities such as swimming are sometimes organised as group activities for particular groups of people such as those expecting a baby, or who have specific health needs such as people with disabilities (see Fig. 1.4).

There are many local clubs which people can join. The Citizen's Advice Bureau is very good at providing information about existing clubs, as are local free newspapers.

People who are not employed because of the economic climate, disability or retirement may wish to learn new skills and expand their knowledge. Many people of different ages have ambitions to learn or to do something which they have not previously had the opportunity to do. It is important to enable and encourage people to work towards achieving their ambitions, hopes and aspirations, however unrealistic or unambitious they may seem to you.

PERSONAL HYGIENE

Another important part of a balanced lifestyle includes maintaining good standards of hygiene. You will see from Activity 1 that maintaining personal and dental hygiene (including visiting the dentist) were included in the list of ways in which we attempt to maintain our health.

Activity 7

 Ask a parent with a small child how they maintain the personal and dental hygiene of the child.
Compare the standard of hygiene for the small child with your own standards.

COMMENT

ⓘ Most people carry out regular hygiene practices automatically; e.g. hand washing after every visit to the toilet.

Hand and foot care

Hand-washing after going to the toilet or after playing with pets, protects us from disease. Inadequate hand-washing after using the toilet can cause diarrhoea and sickness. Bacteria which are present in the intestines and passed out of the body, can be transferred

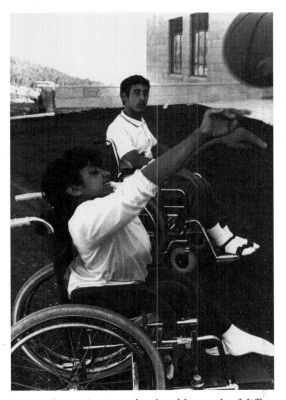

Figure 1.4   *Sport can be played by people of different abilities and disabilities*

from the fingers to the mouth, if hands are not washed properly.

These bacteria are helpful in one part of the body, the bowel or intestine, but are dangerous in other parts such as the mouth and stomach.

There are many other serious diseases which may be passed on from each other, from pets to humans and from insects to humans (see Fig. 1.5). The important point to remember is that routine hygiene practices such as hand-washing protect yourself and others.

Consider how many people could be affected by one person, who works in the kitchen of a café or a restaurant. A person who does not wash their hands (whether they have been to the toilet or not) before

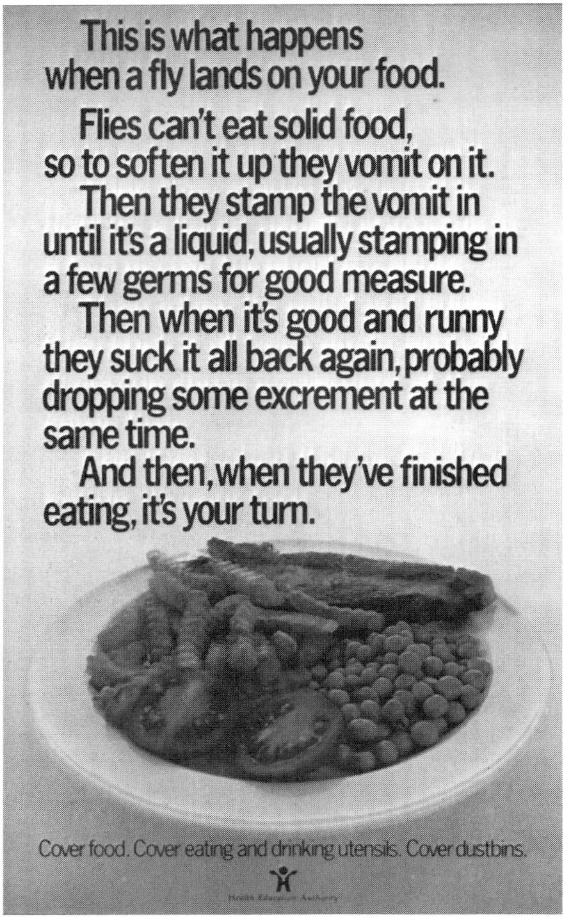

This is what happens when a fly lands on your food.

Flies can't eat solid food, so to soften it up they vomit on it.

Then they stamp the vomit in until it's a liquid, usually stamping in a few germs for good measure.

Then when it's good and runny they suck it all back again, probably dropping some excrement at the same time.

And then, when they've finished eating, it's your turn.

Cover food. Cover eating and drinking utensils. Cover dustbins.

Health Education Authority

Figure 1.5   *Beware of flies in the kitchen!*
Reproduced with permission of the Health Education Authority

preparing food, is likely to cause illness amongst many people. It is also important for food handlers to ensure that they receive medical attention for any cuts or wounds on their hands, that they are properly covered by approved dressings and if advised, to wear protective gloves or not handle food until the wound is healed. These simple precautions may not only prevent ill-health, but may also prevent frail or sick people and small children from developing a fatal illness.

Hand and foot nail care is also important, as dirt and debris may collect under the nails and cause infection. Nails need regular cleaning, which may be done with a soft nail brush during handwashing, or with a nail file or emery board. It is easier to cut nails when they are soft (i.e. during bathing and washing). Nails should be cut across, following the nail shape, and not below the top of the finger or toe. It is often very soothing to massage the hands and feet with a simple skin or hand lotion.

Body care

A small child will probably be given a good wash every day. This would mean either having a shower, bath or a strip wash, ensuring that the most sweaty areas (under the arms and the crotch) are washed, dried and perhaps powdered with a little talc. A small child who is not yet toilet-trained may be washed every time the nappy is changed, to prevent nappy rash. Such frequent washing is not necessary for adults; a daily wash is adequate.

Clothes need to be washed regularly. The child will probably wear clean clothes daily, particularly at an age where it is crawling, feeding itself, falling over and playing outdoors. Clean clothes are very important during hot weather, or where strenuous and dirty occupations and hobbies are undertaken. Clothes absorb perspiration (sweat) and may smell even when the body is clean. This may be unpleasant for everyone.

Hair care

The child's hair may be washed at least once a week, depending on how active it is and what sort of play facilities are generally used.

People wash their hair in different ways and at different times. Certain racial groups use different shampoos, oils and combs. Some groups observe particular customs which restrict hair washing at certain times for specific cultural beliefs and reasons. People with greasy hair may wash it daily, or two or three times a week, while others with dry hair will wash it less often. So depending upon whom you talk to, you will discover that there is a wide variety of hygiene practices and there is no single right way.

Some adult males may shave daily or twice daily, depending upon the speed of growth of the beard. Others may prefer to grow a beard, shaving only in areas of the face which improve the shape of the beard.

Mouth care

How did the parents of the small child maintain the child's dental health in Activity 7? You may have found that when the child was a baby, they did not give it sweet, syrupy drinks, preferring plain boiled water to quench thirst. Even when babies are small, sweet drinks may affect the growing teeth.

Once a small tooth has erupted, it needs to be gently brushed with a soft toothbrush at least twice a day. The parent can create a game from this ritual which the child may enjoy, but if it is not too keen, it may like to play with a toothbrush to get to know it, and maybe even attempt to clean its own teeth. However, children are not very skilful at undertaking tooth care thoroughly, so it is best undertaken or supervised carefully by a parent.

As the child gets older and more teeth erupt, the parents should introduce it to the dentist and take the child for regular check-ups. Fluoride treatment or fluoride tablets may be recommended as a preventive measure to protect the new teeth from decay and for the development of permanent teeth. Both sets of teeth are extremely important. Damaged baby teeth can create problems for the later permanent teeth.

Activity 8

Find out from your local dentist whether fluoride supplements are recommended in your area for babies and small children. You could also find out the natural fluoride content of the local water supply.

COMMENT

Fluoride is a natural mineral found in larger quantities in the water of some areas and in very small traces in others. It protects teeth, which is why it is added to toothpaste and why dentists sometimes coat teeth with it.

The dentist will be aware of the fluoride levels in the water supply and will be able to recommend the appropriate amount of fluoride to be given to babies and small children. The dentist will also be able to advise as to whether or not children should use toothpaste containing fluoride at the same time as fluoride drops or tablets. Too much fluoride will damage the teeth. Because small children are not very good at spitting toothpaste out, the dentist may advise that toothpaste without fluoride is used while the fluoride drops or tablets are being given.

Eating sweets and drinking flavoured drinks such as orange juice should be

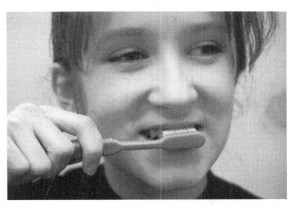

Figure 1.6   *Daily brushing can prevent tooth decay*

restricted to mealtimes, with toothbrushing at least twice a day. The use of fluoride supplements for children and fluoride toothpaste together with regular dental check-ups and necessary treatments, will protect their teeth and gums, and keep them healthy.

People without their own teeth need to brush their gums, cleaning between the cheek and the tooth ridge. Swilling cold water around the mouth helps to remove debris and prevent infection. Dentures need to be brushed regularly and checked to ensure that they fit properly, otherwise food will be difficult to eat and a balanced diet will not be maintained.

Summary

Personal hygiene is important as it ensures that every effort is made to keep the body clean and protected from disease. Your personal hygiene also protects others from disease and it makes you feel good. When your hair is clean and shiny, when you are confident in your smile because your teeth are clean and your gums healthy, when you have eaten and slept well and when you have good relationships with others, you feel good.

Presenting advice

When you want to help others make changes in their lifestyle so that they too will feel better, it is important to remember that we are all different. We all like different foods and have different tastes and cultures; we like different kinds of activities including sports, leisure and recreation; we all may take care of our bodies in different ways, using showers, baths, oils and soaps; we take care of our clothes in different ways. When giving advice to others, it is essential to make sure that it is appropriate to their needs, given the differences mentioned above.

ASSESSING HEALTH PRACTICES

The following activity helps you to appreciate the importance of being able to compare your own health practices with a baseline, and then to determine for yourself which changes you can and want to make. Enabling people to take control of changes which they can manage is an important part of giving health advice to others.

Activity 9

Write down in a notebook everything and every time you eat and drink over a one week period.

When you have done this, compare it with the advice given in the sections 'A balanced diet' and 'Alcohol, tobacco and health'.

COMMENT

Did you find that on some days you had more foods from some food groups than others, but on the whole you ate a balanced diet, or were there any foods which you ate too often and others which you were not eating often enough? Do you need to make changes? What will the changes mean to you in terms of extra effort? Is there enough information to help you?

Did you find that you drank enough fluids in comparison with the recommended amount? Was your alcohol intake below or above the recommended amount over the week?

Did you find it easy or difficult to keep a diary in this way? Was it helpful to you?

Advice

Some professionals recommend keeping diaries for special purposes such as diet or sleep analysis, because it gives a good picture of what is happening over a short period of time. It is easy to forget what we have eaten or drunk from one day to the next. We may feel we are getting a balanced diet, but find that we are not getting enough food from one food group. This may in the long term have a bad effect on our health.

Making a record through keeping a diary, is a method that people can use to assess their own lifestyle. You are then in a better position to discuss with them any changes which they may be able to make. You can use the guidelines from the Health Education Authority, given earlier as a basis for advice.

There are other important documents which contain advice. These include the government recommendations found in the Committee on Medical Aspects of Food Policy (1995) COMA Report.

Activity 10

Having looked at your own and other people's lifestyles, write down as many things as possible which you and others need information about in order to make 'healthy' choices about food, smoking, alcohol, sleep, rest and recreation.

Rearrange your list in the correct order in which this information should be given when advising a client.

Discuss your list (which is now becoming a plan) with other people, to find out what their opinions are.

COMMENT

This activity should have given you a list of important information, arranged in a 'user-friendly' order. This list might contain information about how much exercise we need to keep healthy; what sort of exercise is best for people at different age groups; what the different food groups are and what constitutes a balanced diet. It might also contain how much fluid is recommended daily and the limits for alcohol consumption for men and women. Smokers might like to know how to give up and what sort of help is available locally. It is important to present your advice carefully, as information on all these different aspects of lifestyle, given at the same time, would probably make someone 'switch off'; it may not all be of interest to someone at that point in time.

Information changes over time. It is vital to make sure that any advice you do give is up-to-date. This can be done through regular reading of reports, articles, documents and books on the subjects before giving advice.

Activity 11

From the local Yellow Pages or telephone directory, find out where the local health promotion or health education department is, or where the local health clinics are situated. Go and browse through the health education leaflets on display about any one subject which is of interest to you.

Collect a range of leaflets on this one subject and read each carefully. Make notes about whether you think there is too much information provided or too little to meet your needs.

- Is the language used easy to understand and written in short, easy-to-follow sentences?
- Is there anything which you would like to know which is not included?

Compare the information provided with the list you produced in Activity 10, if it is on a similar subject. Assess whether or not the information addresses the needs of a person with disabilities, either in terms of its presentation e.g. large print, or in terms of its content or resource lists.

COMMENT

 Did you find that the written materials

- were clear

- contained plain English

- used non-sexist language

- were sensitive to cultural and race differences

- used diagrams, charts and other forms of illustration in order to convey clear and usable information?

It is sometimes difficult to make health education materials which address all needs. It may be more effective to identify a target group and address the information specifically at them as more general information would lead to lengthy and irrelevant reading.

In a recent health education publication, Ewles and Simnett (1995) recommend a 'Gobbledygook Test' which measures readability. Take another look at the leaflets from Activity 11. The test asks you to undertake the following:

1 Count a 100 word sample.
2 Count the number of complete sentences in this sample.
3 Count the total number of words in a complete sentence.
4 Divide the number of words by the num-

ber of sentences. This gives you the average sentence length.
5 Count the number of words with three or more syllables in the 100 words. This gives the percentage of long words in the sample (numbers and symbols are counted as short words; hyphenated words are counted as two words).
6 Add the average sentence length to the percentage of long words to give the test score; the higher the score the lower the 'readability'.

Well written and well presented materials are a useful resource in health education.

COLLECTING INFORMATION FOR HEALTH PROMOTION

You need to find out what is important to individuals before giving them any advice. Talking to them, assessing their needs, finding out what they already know, undertaking observations, reviewing records and discussing needs with colleagues helps to provide a rounded picture on how to proceed. When you have undertaken this assessment, you may then select the area which is of most interest to your target group at that point in time. This fits into the assessment stage of Table 1.2 below.

The next stage is the *planning* stage, which means you need to think about the best way of sharing this information. There are many different ways of sharing information with people either on a one-to-one basis or in a group. An example would be simply *discussing* it, talking it over with each other. However, it is well known that we do not always remember everything we hear and discuss. Therefore some other ways of sharing

Table 1.2:   Methods of promoting physical exercise

Aim	Possible methods
Health awareness or consciousness of benefits of exercise	Mass media, talks, displays, campaigns, leaflets, programmes, videos, group work, promotions, invitations etc. which highlight the benefits of exercise to people of different age groups and at different life-stages and abilities
Improving knowledge, providing information	Teaching, lectures, reading materials, educational videos, displays and exhibitions, library visits, project work aimed at target such as elderly people attending a day centre, small children at a play group, pregnant women or people with disabilities
Social change, changing the social environment	Working with target group such as older people and with leisure centre manager in order to obtain a change in physical leisure centre policy to be sensitive to their needs. Broadening the image of leisure centre users to include people with special needs and thus encourage use. Working with parents to obtain safer surfaces under children's play equipment in local park.
Behaviour change, changing the lifestyle of individuals	Exercise groups, support for people who have specific health needs such as people who have had a hip replacement or other disabilities. Exchange of ideas for improving exercise regimes. Problem-solving discussions using case-studies or real examples from people in the group.
Self-awareness, improving self-esteem and decision-making	Informal groupwork with target group. Discussion on one-to-one basis or in groups regarding whether or not to undertake exercise programmes. Exploring reasons which prevent participation.

information may be needed to enable people to recall, test their knowledge, and remind themselves of what has been discussed, when you are no longer around to help them.

Health education leaflets and handouts are the most common ways in which information can be given, taken away and studied later. These may be made by you and so adapted to the people you are working with, or may be produced by a variety of organisations.

Other methods include diagrams, pic-tures, tape-recordings, videos, photographs, quizzes which may be multiple choice, mod-els, the 'real' thing (e.g. glasses with the actual units of alcohol), stories, poems, com-puter programs or games.

Activity 12

The next time you are in a learning situation, make a note of the different ways in which you are taught and which you enjoy most. Jot down the different methods

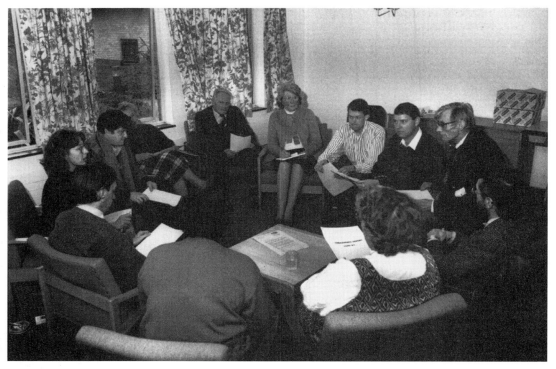

Figure 1.7   *Group discussion can be an enjoyable and effective way of learning*

teachers use to help you to learn and include a note beside each method indicating your level of involvement.

COMMENT

ⓘ Some methods of communicating or teaching have a high level of involvement, while others require you to do very little. Some enable you to participate and share your knowledge; others require you to be fairly passive.

High level of involvement	Low level of involvement
Discussions	National/local press and TV
Brainstorm	Billboard advertising
Trial and error	Lecture
Role play	Displays

Project work	Leaflets and other reading materials
Visits	Videos and computer exercises
Interactive computer programs and games	

These are just a few of the possible ways in which health teaching may be undertaken. When you are planning for health education, you need to think about your own comfort as well as the comfort of those for whom your efforts are intended. Do you feel comfortable doing all the talking or listening? Do you feel comfortable when everyone present has an opportunity to join in? You also need to think about the aims of your health education when you are considering the possible methods. Ewles and Simnett (1995) suggest five main aims of health promotion with accompanying methods to suit these: health awareness; improving knowledge; social and environmental change; behaviour change; and self-awareness. If we take the health promotion example of physical exercise and look at these five aims, we can see some similarities and some differences in possible methods; see Table 1.2 on page 21.

While it is possible to consider each of these aims separately as we have above, you will see that there is likely to be some overlap.

Activity 13

Using the five aims outlined above, look at a specific issue such as home safety, exercise and school children, nutrition or another health promotion topic, and identify the most appropriate methods for each.

COMMENT

Working for a change in the physical or social environment, such as improving children's play areas, means that those involved will need to have in-depth knowledge about the potential risks. Their knowledge will therefore improve, as will their self-awareness, lifestyle etc.

Activity 14

Read the chapter on *Teaching and Learning* from Ewles and Simnett (1995) (or a similar chapter from an appropriate book on health promotion – see resource list at the end of this chapter) which should be available in the library.

COMMENT

You will have learned that there are several ways in which health education information can be communicated depending upon your approach. You will

need to think about the best methods for your *target* audience. There is no right or wrong way, and you will find out what works well and what does not by talking to people and asking them what they thought of the video, quiz etc. If a method does not go down too well, it may be that it is wrong for your group but might work well with another. People seem to remember more where they have been able to participate rather than simply receive information.

The process of thinking about lifestyle and making 'healthy' changes can be seen in a problem-solving cycle in Fig. 1.8 on page 24. Using this cycle to guide you in planning health education activities may contribute to your success and may also draw attention to areas which need to change to build on your success. You will probably change your approach as you get *feedback* from people, and this is why the problem-solving cycle is an important one to remember. The feedback or *evaluation* forms part of the *assessment* before recommencing health promotion activities.

It is very important to think about the ways in which you will find out whether people make any changes to their lifestyle following the information you have given. This may be done by:

- keeping their names and telephone numbers and phoning them at an agreed date.

- organising another group meeting and discussing their progress and any barriers to them being able to make any changes.

It is worth bearing in mind that people may not have changed their lifestyle straight away. People often need to wait until the time is 'right' for them before taking action, so it doesn't necessarily mean that your efforts were wasted if they have not made changes straight away.

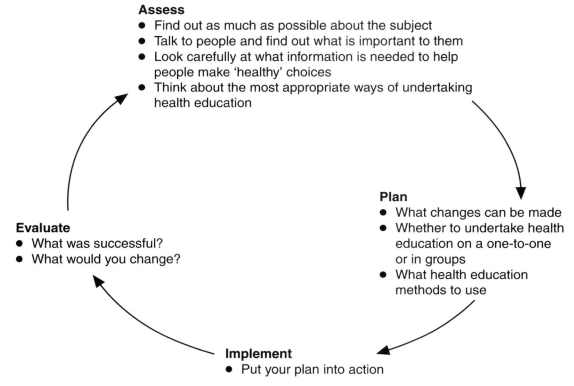

Assess
- Find out as much as possible about the subject
- Talk to people and find out what is important to them
- Look carefully at what information is needed to help people make 'healthy' choices
- Think about the most appropriate ways of undertaking health education

Plan
- What changes can be made
- Whether to undertake health education on a one-to-one or in groups
- What health education methods to use

Evaluate
- What was successful?
- What would you change?

Implement
- Put your plan into action

Figure 1.8   *A problem-solving cycle*

Activity 15

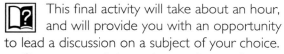 This final activity will take about an hour, and will provide you with an opportunity to lead a discussion on a subject of your choice.

- Get a group of about six people together and ask each one to talk about a home accident they have experienced and how they dealt with it.
- Find out what skills or knowledge they would have liked to have had before the event in order to prevent the accident occurring or during the event to enable them to deal with the situation.

COMMENT

ℹ You probably found that everyone in turn was able to talk about an accident and have views on either prevention and treatment or both. They might have wanted prior knowledge which would have enabled them to reduce hazards, or they might have wanted first aid knowledge and skills. They might have attributed the cause to environmental hazards for which they are not responsible and therefore wish that somebody had 'done something' to reduce risks, suggesting a social change aim for health promotion.

You have now led a group discussion on a health promotion issue and probably can see the potential for running a group which has a high level of involvement of each group member. The group members may have learned from each other and you may have identified a need to organise further sessions where first aid is the topic, and someone skilled and trained in the area leads the group.

Thus health promotion may be on-going, with the first discussion leading on to other activities. It may involve other people with different skills and knowledge, and lead to different actions being undertaken by the target group.

SUMMARY

So far, this chapter has asked you to examine your lifestyle and the lifestyles of other people. It has emphasised that we are individuals and have different needs, cultures, preferences; this should be respected when health education is undertaken. Individuals often have some knowledge of health education and may already be taking measures to keep themselves healthy. This also needs to be taken into account when presenting health information to others. It is important to give praise for every effort that people make, as well as giving advice on those areas about which they know little.

Finding out what people know and what they want to know is an essential part of the assessment process. Selecting ways in which advice can be best provided, and working out methods for getting feedback on the effectiveness of the advice is also necessary. You should now have a good idea about the advice which is needed for some aspects of a healthy lifestyle, and where to obtain further information. Facts are constantly changing as new information comes to light. It is essential that you keep an eye on the media and on new books and articles, to ensure that your advice is up-to-date.

References and resources

Ewles, L., Simnett, I. (1995), *Promoting Health. A Practical Guide.* 3rd Edition, Scutari Press, London.

Hubley, J. (1993), *Communicating Health. An action guide to health education and health promotion.* Macmillan Press Ltd., London.

Kemm, J., Close, A. (1995), *Health Promotion. Theory and Practice.* Macmillan, London.

Kiger, A. M. (1995), *Teaching for Health,* 2nd edition. Churchill Livingstone, Singapore.

Pike, S., Forster, D. (1995), *Health Promotion for All.* Churchill Livingstone, London.

The Health Education Authority, Hamilton House, Mabledon Place, London, WC1 H9CX.

Reducing the risk of injury

HAZARDS WHICH AFFECT HEALTH

In order to look at hazards which may affect the health of individuals and any actions we might take to reduce risk of injury from such hazards, let us firstly divide the section into possible areas where hazards may occur and the groups of individuals at greatest risk.

Accidents are a major cause of ill-health, injuries and death, and affect all age groups. Those especially vulnerable include children, young adults, older people, and any person with reduced physical or mental capacity. In this section we consider safety in the home environment, on the roads, the work environment, the local and social environment. The government's document, Health of the Nation, set targets for reducing accidents, illness, disability and even deaths resulting directly from accidents.

Activity 16

Obtain access to the part of the Health of the Nation document dealing with accidents. Are there any results to report yet on how accident prevention is being carried out, and with what effect?

Note: This information may not be readily available, and you may need to ask your tutor to direct you.

PROMOTING A SAFE ENVIRONMENT

The environment greatly affects the health and quality of our lives. Factors affecting health may not always directly involve your client's choice, e.g. environmental hygiene (clean water, safe sewage disposal), atmospheric pollution, even housing. Promoting a safe environment for clients, colleagues and self should be one of your many functions. This helps to improve and maintain the health of the nation.

In order to achieve as safe an environment as possible, it is important that you are able to recognise a potentially harmful situation. This might best be achieved by being aware of people who are especially at risk. We have already stated that all individuals are at risk and we are aware of the higher risk groups; but consider people who are depressed, bereaved, physically ill, people with reduced hearing or sight and those whose cultures may encourage differing opinions from our own. Environmental awareness begins shortly after birth, continuing throughout life. These people may not have the same awareness/control as you would have. You must be extra vigilant in recognising potential dangers and promoting your client's and their carer's awareness and adaptability towards the avoidance of those dangers.

PROTECTING YOURSELF

As a carer you will share responsibility with other staff, keeping your clients in a safe environment. You also hold a level of responsibility for yourself, maintaining safe working practice, in whatever environment. When dealing with health emergencies it is important to work safely, protecting yourself from injury/infection. Do not risk injury to yourself (e.g. following a client's electrical shock or road traffic accident).

Preventing back injury

There is a recognised high rate of back injury amongst carers. Your employer will provide training to make sure that you are able to lift safely, in accordance with European Union regulations. Always lift with equipment, if available, or lift/turn with another person. Changing beds or cleaning incontinent people in the night can pose problems, so try to make sure that these actions are done by two people. It is safer for both you and your clients. If a client is falling or slipping, do not injure yourself in trying to prevent this. Allow him/her to slide slowly and gently to the ground without causing undue damage to either of you.

Basic principles of safe lifting

Always lift with equipment or another carer. Decide upon a plan of action and who will issue leading commands. Choose the lift that will be safest and most comfortable for your client and then you should:

1 Explain to your client how you are going to lift him/her.
2 Clear obstacles and ensure brakes are applied to beds/wheelchairs.
3 Provide privacy and ask the client to help as much as they can.
4 Ensure the distance you are going to lift is as short as possible. If you do not feel confident about the lift, do not attempt it.
5 Stand as close as possible to your client, making sure you have a firm, comfortable hold in them.
6 Keeping your back straight but not rigid, position your feet with the leading foot pointing in the direction you will be mov-

ing. Move your feet while you are turning to avoid back strain.
7 Use your hips, knees and body weight to lift by lowering yourself to your client's level and using your legs to take strain. The leader should give commands so that you all co-operate together.

Scenario

Mrs Caldwell is an overweight 74-year-old living in a residential home. She is blind and relies heavily on carers to assist her in many of the activities of daily life. In spite of this she remains cheerful and likes to maintain the little independence she has. She does not like asking for help or to be a nuisance to carers.

She has asked you to help her to the bathroom for a wash before going to bed. Once there she asks you if you would assist her in having a bath. You notice that somebody has borrowed the slip mat and portable bath hoist. Time is against you and Mrs Caldwell is encouraging you to proceed, insisting that you will manage.

Having been unexpectedly asked to assist with bathing, you may proceed to bath without equipment, risking injury to yourself or the client, or you may help her to sit down, wrapped in a warm towel, and fetch the equipment and slip mat. You have four other clients to assist with bathing and time is against you.

Activity 17

 What action would you take? Why? How do you think Mrs Caldwell might feel if you insist on fetching the equipment? What explanations would you give her?

List some of the points on safe lifting you should consider when making your decision.

COMMENT

It is hoped that you would explain to Mrs Caldwell that you would be happy to assist her in bathing but in order to not risk injury either to her, or to yourself, while lifting, you would take a short time to fetch the portable hoist. While doing so you would make sure she was safely seated and warmly wrapped in a towel. Remembering that as Mrs Caldwell never liked to appear to be a nuisance you would need to reassure her that fetching the equipment was not a problem to you. You are not trying to reduce her sense of dignity or reduce her power in making her own decisions.

Points you might consider when making your decision:

- You would need client co-operation

- If you do not feel confident about the lift do not attempt it

- Always lift with equipment (or another carer) if available

- Choose the lift that will be safest and most comfortable for your client and you.

Blood and body fluids

When dealing with blood and body fluids your employer has guidelines (Universal Precautions) to work within, to protect you and other staff from the risk of infections, in particular Hepatitis B and the HIV virus. These are carried in blood and can be passed on through cuts in the skin, so protect any cuts you have with waterproof dressings. Also, take care if you have an open skin complaint like eczema. You should be provided with seamless disposable vinyl gloves and disposable aprons when dealing with body fluids.

Spillages should be dealt with within policy guidelines, but this is not always possible in an emergency situation. If they are able, show the injured person how to apply pressure themselves to a bleeding wound. If you need to apply pressure and gloves are unavailable make sure you use lots of absorbent material, e.g. towels. If you come into contact with blood you should wash the affected area in running water for at least 10 minutes and report the incident to qualified staff who will advise you of the safety guidelines to follow.

DANGERS IN THE HOME

A person's home may be where they live with their family/carers or it may be a residential or nursing homes, private or state-financed. Residential or nursing homes are bound by strict guidelines, set both externally and internally, with regard to the health and safety of all individuals either residing there, working or visiting. In contrast, the safety of a family home depends on family members and visitors, and their awareness of potential hazards and general common sense.

Thousands of people are injured in their home every year as a result of burns/scalds, cuts, suffocation/choking, falls, drowning, poisonous substances and electrocution. These accidents are often the result of:

- incorrectly used/stored potentially dangerous hazardous substances
- inadequate or faulty equipment
- poor design of accommodation

High risk groups of individuals have been identified, but even so most accidents could be prevented by forward thinking and common sense.

Floors

Make sure there are no loose or worn carpets where people can catch their feet and trip or fall: this applies especially to stair carpets. Avoid loose mats and rugs, especially on highly polished floors. Ensure that floors are not slippery when wet; in residential homes, place markers to warn of potential hazards. Wear non-slip shoes as appropriate. Wipe up any spillages immediately. Do not trail electrical flexes across floors and doorways. Ensure adequate lighting. Do not leave toys etc. scattered about on floors.

Surfaces

Preferably keep children out of the kitchen when cooking but certainly keep them away from the cooker and always use a cooker guard. Do not allow pan handles to stick out over the edge of the cooker and never leave a chip pan unattended. Do not leave sharp tools or cooking implements where a child may reach them. Make sure that toddlers cannot reach hot dishes on the table or work surfaces and are not able to tug on table-cloths.

Poisonous substances

When buying potentially hazardous substances (cleaning agents etc.), try to ensure that they have childproof tops, and always store them in a cupboard with a childproof fastener (preferably a locked cupboard and one that is fixed high on the wall). Keep any alcoholic drinks in locked or childproof cupboards, as it is very tempting for toddlers and young children to experiment with alcoholic

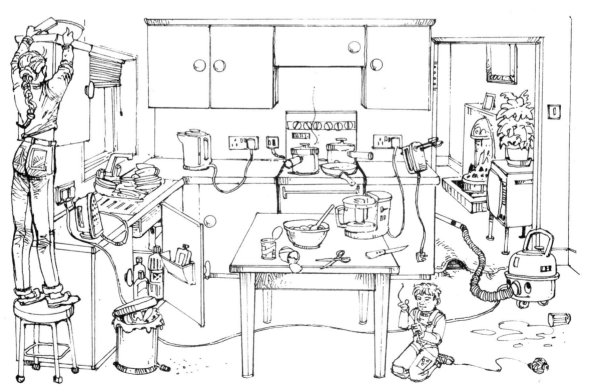

Figure 1.9   *Can you count the number of potential hazards in this kitchen?*

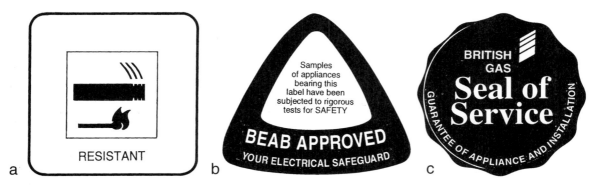

Figure 1.10   *(a) flame resistant symbol, (b) electrical safety symbol, (c) gas safety symbol*

drinks. Any medicines should have child-proof openings and should be out of reach from toddlers, preferably in a locked cupboard. Take out-of-date medication to a chemist's shop, where they can dispose of it safely; do not throw it down the sink or toilet, or throw into general rubbish bins.

Electrics/gas

Ensure that electrical appliances are well maintained, and only plugged in while in use. Portable heaters should also be well maintained and not moved while hot or in use. Fire-guards should be used and safely fixed; this advice is not just for toddlers, but also for elderly or infirm people. Plants and flowers should not be kept on top of the television in case water comes into contact with the electrical circuit. Electric blankets should be unplugged before getting into bed. Switch off bedside lamps before going to sleep. Do not use electrical appliances in a bathroom. Ensure that gas water heaters are adequately maintained and have adequate ventilation when in use: never cover air bricks.

Falls

Use a stool when trying to reach an object from a cupboard or shelf. Do not over-reach, and try to install cupboards within normal reach. If toddlers are around, use a safety gate at the top and bottom of a flight of stairs. Fix two non-slip handrails on the staircase for elderly or infirm people to ease going up or down the stairs. In extreme cases of frailty or disability consider a stairlift. Teach children how to use stairs safely. In case of falls, have safety glass fitted in internal doors. Keep items of furniture away from windows, even on ground level. Children are keen to explore, so never leave a child alone near an open window, however close to the ground you are. It may even be necessary to have bars fitted at windows, though these should be removable in case of fire. Check that cots are safe. For elderly or infirm people it may be advised to have grab-rails fitted round the bath, shower or toilet, and non-slip mats in the bath. Grab rails may also be usefully fitted on entrance steps and rooms where there may be steps leading from one to another.

Lacerations

Do not leave any sharp objects/instruments where a child may reach them. If a child is old enough and capable of using scissors, ensure that they are round ended and that the child is supervised and not allowed to walk around carrying them. Keep breakable ornaments out of children's reach: not only may they break the ornament, but they may then cut themselves on the broken pieces. Do not leave razors or loose blades lying around: dispose of loose blades in empty cans or if in a residential home, you may use an official disposal bin.

Do not use cracked or chipped crockery: not only will these items harbour germs, but they will shatter easily when in use or when being washed.

Burns/scalds

We have already identified precautions to take when cooking, but always remember to use a strong pair of oven gloves when handling hot pans and dishes. As previously mentioned, protect all fires with fire-guards, keeping matches and lighters out of reach. Remember to check ashtrays before going to bed and do not be tempted to smoke in bed. Always check that food and drinks you administer are not too hot: this ranges from a baby's feeding bottle to assisting a disabled adult or elderly person. Do not use an unprotected hot water bottle in a baby's bed. Do not dry or air clothes near an open fire or overnight storage heater. Nightwear should be composed of non-inflammable materials. Aerosol canisters should be kept away from heat and should never be punctured or burned even when empty.

Always ensure that bath water is of a safe temperature for babies, children and adults and do not leave them unsupervised: scalds are easily caused by adding water from the hot tap, and it is also very easy to drown in a small amount of bath water.

Choking/asphyxiation

It is advisable that babies and young children are not left unsupervised when eating and drinking, as they are particularly vulnerable to choking. Children under the age of three should not be allowed to play with small objects: they are always tempted to place items in their mouths and this easily leads to choking. Babies and young children should not be sleeping on soft pillows, as they are liable to asphyxiation. When a baby has been fed remove any bibs (especially the plastic backed ones) before placing back into the cot; it is better not to lie them flat too soon after a meal. Babies should be laid on their side and not on their front. Children should not be allowed to play with ribbon or string unless supervised, as they can easily choke on these. Plastic bags should never be used in play and should be stored safely in the house: these are difficult to remove when placed over the face.

Activity 18

You can carry out this activity either during work experience, or else in your own home.

Choose an area other than the kitchen, e.g. hall, staircase, passage, landing, living room, bedroom, bathroom, garden. Bear in mind the specific needs of the people who use this area (i.e. clients in a residential home, your family, etc.), and make a list of the specific safety precautions you need to follow.

AVOIDING HAZARDS IN THE GARDEN

This area may be divided into hazards for children, and for adults working in the garden.

Children at play

Young children should not play outdoors unsupervised. Always keen to explore, they will look for gaps in fences, hedges and gates. Ensure that all paths and boundaries are safe and in good repair: fix childproof locks on gates so they will not rush out onto the road.

Even after these precautions your garden may be hazardous. If pets are kept, make sure that all excrement is cleared from the garden daily, as this may harbour worms and more serious germs. Make sure that all garden tools are safely locked away: not only will children be at risk of falling or cutting themselves on them but they will be quite happy to use them as new toys and may cause harm to other children. Any garden chemicals (e.g. weed killers, rat poisons, slug pellets) should also be kept under lock and key. The garden should be cleared of any dangerous items such as broken glass or rusty nails. If there are wells, ponds, water butts these should be safely covered.

Do not allow children to play with catapults, bows and arrows etc., until you are sure they are old enough and responsible. Young children should be discouraged from running around with sharp toys in their mouths: these may cause serious cuts if the children fall and perforate the roof of the mouth. Discourage children from eating plants and weeds: some may be poisonous, and could make the children very ill. Older children love experimenting with lighting fires, but do not allow them to play in the garden with matches, and keep them away from fireworks on Bonfire night.

Adults at work

Adults should be advised to wear sturdy shoes when gardening to avoid any injuries with sharp gardening tools. When mowing lawns, clear any loose stones from the grass before starting, so that stones do not fly up through and out of the mower, causing injury either to themselves or to any bystanders. Electric mowers should be dis-

connected after use. If it is a petrol mower, do not smoke while refilling the petrol tank. All power tools should have loose cables kept out of reach and looped over the shoulder: cables should be kept away from bladed instruments. Any garden fires should be put out before night and should not be left unattended.

General hazards

Anybody who has been playing or working in the garden should be encouraged to wash their hands when returning indoors. People are vulnerable to tetanus germs if they are outdoors playing or working with the soil, especially children with cuts and grazes or adults with rose-thorn puncture wounds. Check your client's tetanus status: if they are up to date with immunisations they are less vulnerable to any dangers.

Anybody outdoors in sunny weather should be aware of the dangers of overexposure to the sun, burning and skin cancer. Do not encourage outdoor activity when the sun is at its strongest (around midday).

Remember *Slip, Slap, Slop*: Slip on a t-shirt, slap on a hat, slop on a high protection sun cream, before going outside.

SAFETY ON THE ROADS

Outside the home, road accidents are the most common form of danger. If people behaved more responsibly towards others and took more responsibility for their own safety, there would be fewer accidents.

Car safety

Drivers should stick to speed limits. Many accidents can be prevented if the car is not driven above the speed limit. In hazardous weather conditions (such as fog, ice, snow), travel by road should be avoided unless absolutely necessary. Cars should not be driven by people who are under age or do not hold a current driving licence. If somebody is sick, feels ill or tired they will have difficulty in concentrating, and so should not drive. Certain drugs, therapeutic or otherwise, may have an effect on driving: alcohol in particular impairs the driver's ability and reactions. Accidents can be caused by the driver having poor eyesight; being emotionally disturbed, depressed, sad or angry; being distracted by passengers (people talking, children chattering or playing, even animals that are not well behaved in cars). Having a deadline to meet can cause a driver to be too close to the car in front and may cause lack of concentration. The driver may also take risks which he or she would otherwise not take, especially overtaking. Drivers need to be familiar with the Highway Code. The number of passengers should not exceed the limit of the size of the car.

Activity 19

In groups, make a list of recent government campaigns to prevent road accidents (e.g. through drinking and driving, or from driving too fast). Discuss which one you think is most effective, and why.

SEAT BELTS

All passengers are required by law to wear seat belts. Every year as many as 6,000 children are passengers involved in car accidents and approximately 120 of these are killed. Babies and all children should be seated in appropriately sized car seats, secured by standard seat belts or strapped in using seat belts, and preferably seated in the back of the car. All items used should carry the British

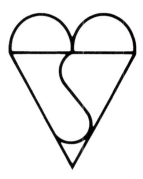

Figure 1.11   *The BSI Kitemark is awarded when the product has been made to the correct British Standard*

Standard Kitemark to show the approval of the British Standards Institute (see Fig. 1.11).

Care should be taken not to trap fingers in car doors. These should be ideally fitted with childproof locks and children should be discouraged from leaning against the doors.

Motorcycles

Motorcyclists abide by the same rules as the car driver: the Highway Code. They should be encouraged to enrol on a motorcyclist safety and proficiency course, to receive tuition from experts. A crash helmet bearing the British Standard Kitemark should be worn at all times. This should be replaced if it becomes damaged in any way, as this may render it unsafe. Sensible wear should be considered: preferably leather or decent waterproof gear, or certainly clothes that will keep the biker warm, dry and protect him or her in case of accidents. Road safety applies as with car drivers, but a motorbike is often smaller than a car and not so easily seen; motorcyclists should always make allowances for that, especially when pulling out of junctions or overtaking another vehicle.

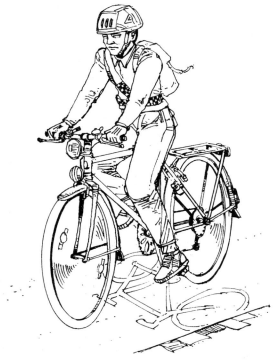

Figure 1.12   *Cyclists should be properly dressed and equipped for cycling in traffic*

Bicycles

Cyclists who are poor road users render themselves unsafe in traffic. As with motorcyclists, cyclists should be advised to learn about safety and enrol on cycling proficiency courses run by schools or local authorities. If a cyclist is unsafe he runs the risk of injuring himself, any pedestrians or other road users. Cycling helmets are not compulsory but have been shown to save lives. Clothing should not be loose, to avoid getting caught in the spokes of the bike or any passing vehicles. If travelling at night, it is advisable to wear a fluorescent sash or bib and to ensure that all lights are in good working order.

Cyclists should understand the Highway Code: they should stay in single file in traffic, keep close to the kerb and give consideration to other road users.

Luggage carried should be kept to a minimum, heavy items might cause the cyclist to have less control of the bike in an emergency. Parents who transport young children on bike seats should take special care.

Pedestrians

Pedestrians should be taught the rules of road safety from an early age: they should stop, look and listen at the kerb before crossing the road. If there is a lollipop lady or an official crossing these should be used, as they are there for our safety. It is not easy to judge distances even if we have good sight and hearing, so it is better to wait if unsure rather than hurry across, fall and be harmed or cause an accident to another person. Any pets should be kept under strict control at all times. At night fluorescent or reflective clothing should be worn and we should stick to paths. Many older children are quite sensible when crossing roads but adults should always set them an example.

HAZARDS IN THE SOCIAL SETTING

Recreation

We have discussed some of the hazards children may face when playing in their own gardens, and some of the skills they need to acquire when walking along paths or crossing roads. Let us look at local playgrounds. The same basic rules apply to children as when playing in their gardens: to be supervised, to ensure the ground is clear, for ponds to be covered, not to play with unsuitable toys, not to eat plants or weeds. It is also essential that all play equipment such as climbing frames, is in good repair. The same applies to the school playground.

School gyms or sports centres should have equipment that is regularly checked and maintained. Teachers or people who have specialist training in the use of the equipment should always be on hand to prevent accident. In sports centres, pools are always supervised by designated people with life saving certificates.

Many social centres and gyms have a bar where clients enjoy a drink afterwards. They might need a reminder of the dangers of drinking and driving, especially after a heavy work-out when they might be very thirsty and feel the need for a higher fluid intake.

HOLIDAYS

A badly planned holiday can be hazardous, whether camping, caravanning or walking. All equipment and modes of transport should be thoroughly checked for usability or signs of wear and tear (this especially applies to activities such as climbing or potholing). It is advisable not to attempt an 'action' holiday unless fully trained or equipped: this applies even to hiking, especially in bad weather.

When camping or caravanning, you should always ensure that precautions are taken with any heaters or cooking stoves, switching off after use, not smoking nearby, having a fire extinguisher handy, ensuring adequate ventilation, not leaving children alone in the van or tent.

On an outdoor holiday, do not drink water unless you are sure that it is safe for drinking, as untreated water can make you very ill. When outdoors, make sure clothing is suitable, especially footwear. Always plan where you are going and if possible, tell

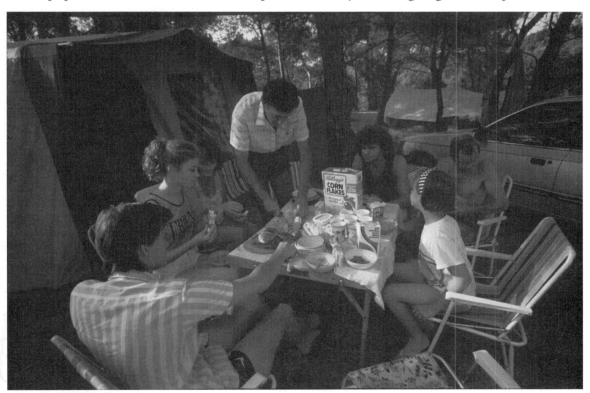

Figure 1.13   *Camping can be fun – but only if proper safety precautions are taken*

somebody. It is preferable not to camp, hike, climb or pot-hole alone. Keep all animals under strict control and follow the Country Code with special regard to litter. Always remember to take a First Aid box.

Work

The Health and Safety at Work Act 1974 provides guidelines for the protection of all employers, employees, self-employed people and the public at large. It aims to protect people against hazards in their working environment.

Accidents may happen to anybody you may work with, especially our 'higher risk' groups, but people who feel unwell or tired are also at risk. Accidents may be caused by those who become careless and rush jobs because they are trying to meet a deadline; any person who has had an emotional upset which caused them to be sad or angry; or people who are under the influence of drugs or alcohol. The Act clearly states the responsibilities of the employers, managers and employees.

EMPLOYERS' DUTIES

1 to provide information, instruction, training, supervision for health and safety at work
2 to provide and maintain safe equipment systems
3 to allow safe use, handling, transport, storage of substances or equipment
4 to ensure the health, safety and welfare of the employer at work.

MANAGERS' DUTIES

1 to provide training for safe working practices
2 to induct all new staff before beginning their work, as to the safe departmental practices and make them aware of hazards in the work environment
3 to ensure all staff adhere to working guidelines
4 to report and record all accidents.

EMPLOYEES' DUTIES

1 to adhere to instructions of equipment operation (use only materials according to recommended procedures)
2 to use protective equipment/clothing as provided
3 not to interfere with or misuse anything for the provisions of health/safety/welfare
4 to comply with requirements imposed by employer
5 to take care of health/safety of self/others.

Let us look briefly at the Control of Substances Hazardous to Health Act (COSHH) 1990. The Act provides advice on ensuring the safety of clients/carers who could be at risk if exposed to harmful or hazardous substances, e.g. those used for cleaning, decorating and pest control. Your employer must comply with these deadlines, thereby not exposing you or your clients to risk if dealing with hazardous substances.

Activity 20

Ask three people you know to check if there are clear health and safety notices displayed in their place of work. If possible, ask them to take photocopies of these notices for you to examine.

Are there any ways in which these notices could be improved, e.g. is any information unclear, or badly presented? Why do you think any possible changes may not already have been implemented?

Design your own health and safety notice for display in your college/school.

LOCAL ENVIRONMENT

Bearing in mind once again our 'higher risk' groups, let us consider the local environment. We have discussed designated play areas, gardens and playgrounds, stating that very young children should be supervised at all times. What about older children, who are allowed to venture off on their own? It is advisable that they inform a parent/carer where they are going, with whom, and when they will be back. Explain to them why somebody should know this information: if they understand the reasons why, they are more likely to adhere to these rules.

Personal safety

Advise children about the dangers of becoming involved with strangers in a way that will not hold them in terror of any person they do not know. Warn them about animals they are not familiar with. Their own pets might be very friendly but other animals might be wary of strangers and especially children if they are not used to them (pets are often frightened by unfamiliar noises).

Water safety

Ideally children should be taught to swim so that if they are tempted to go near water they will be prepared in case of accidents. Canals, ponds, rivers, locks and reservoirs are all sources of danger, not just to children but to older people who may be less agile, if fishing or walking by river banks.

Car parks

We have previously discussed the use of main roads, but car parks hold dangers too. Dodging in and out of stationary cars should not be encouraged, as vehicles may reverse without noticing children playing. It is especially tempting for children to want to explore lorries, so the dangers of climbing onto vehicles should be pointed out.

Derelict buildings and building sites

Young children love exploring: what better play area than derelict buildings, even building sites, especially if the workers have finished for the day? They are greatly at risk in any of these situations. On building sites there may be dangerous equipment which could harm them or their playmates, and they could be at risk of falling while exploring their new play area.

Derelict buildings, old warehouses and even houses may be infested with rats. There may be broken glass about, weakened floorboards, frayed ropes that they might love to swing on. Old factories may have waste products dumped or stored there which could be hazardous to handle. If an accident should happen in a derelict building it may take a lot longer for playmates to summon help. This could be a life-threatening situation where any delay could mean loss of life.

Railway lines

Children should be taught the dangers of playing or going for walks along railway lines. They should be made aware of the risks of lines, bridges, banks, level crossings. This might also apply to elderly or infirm people who, while walking along embankments or disused tracks, might trip or fall, leading to broken limbs or head injuries. Summoning help in an isolated area might not be easy.

Overhead cables can be a danger. If kites become stuck in pylons or cables, it is tempting to climb up and retrieve them, but children may be in serious danger of falling or being electrocuted.

SUMMARY

In spite of strict adherence to national and local policies and use of common sense when dealing with clients in your working environment, accidents will happen, and health emergencies will arise. You are now in a better position to help reduce risk of injury from hazards or hazardous substances. Let us discuss ways of dealing with health emergencies.

Dealing with health emergencies

An emergency situation is not necessarily life-threatening, but should be dealt with effectively. Every emergency is different and each individual should be treated according to the type of injury they suffer. You should act calmly, promptly, and correctly.

An emergency can occur at any time. The cause may be as simple as food blocking the air passage to the lungs (airway), or as complicated as a road traffic accident, either of which could result in a number of problems.

YOUR ROLE AND RESPONSIBILITIES

Over a million people in Britain are treated in hospitals annually from injuries sustained in accidents. Over 6,000 victims of home accidents die – the same number as are involved in road accidents. When working with clients, in any setting, you may have to deal with an emergency situation until help arrives. Let us look at the principles of First Aid: remember that every second counts, and prompt action could save a life.

Your aims are to:

• preserve life
• limit the effects of the condition
• promote recovery

Your responsibilities are to:

1 Remain outwardly calm and confident and assess the situation quickly, without putting yourself, the victim, or others in further danger. Summon appropriate help, perhaps a relative or carer, a qualified member of staff, or the expert help of a doctor or ambulance. Send somebody else for help – do not leave your client.
2 If possible identify the illness or injury which affects your client. Simple observation may help, e.g. looking at skin colour, obvious bleeding, temperature, swelling or distortion of their limbs. If the client is in obvious danger, e.g. from fire, toxic chemicals or an unsafe building, remove them from danger; otherwise do not move them.
3 Administer treatment that may be immediately necessary. Maintain an open *airway* (the breathing passages that lead from the mouth/nose to the lungs). Ensure adequate *breathing*. Maintain *circulation* (the flow of blood through the body). This is the ABC of resuscitation. Providing your client's heart is beating, you may need to place him in the recovery position to keep his airway open and ensure that if he vomits, this drains away from his mouth and he does not choke.

Sending for medical/emergency aid

Although you should always have a senior member of staff working with you, you will be expected to know how to send for emergency aid. Call the General Practitioner (GP) by ringing the surgery or health centre's emergency number. Send for him/her in the case of sudden illness. He/she might ask you to also send for an ambulance when given details of the client's condition. With a serious accident, call directly for an ambulance by dialling the national emergency number, 999. Ensure you always have access to GP's telephone numbers in case of emergencies. Report all accidents to the senior staff and fill in an accident report.

The first aid box
Activity 21

 Discuss in groups of three the following questions:
What is the purpose of a first aid box?
What do you think would make a suitable container?
List what you think are the essential items to keep in it. What would you use these items for?
Where and how would you sensibly store your box?

COMMENT

 Essential items include:

- 10 individually wrapped sterile adhesive dressings
- 1 sterile eye pad
- 1 triangular bandage
- 1 sterile covering for a serious wound
- 6 safety pins

- 3 medium sized sterile dressings
- 1 large sterile dressing
- 1 extra large sterile dressing

Extras might be:

- extra triangular bandages
- packs of sterile cotton wool
- tweezers
- scissors
- a thermometer
- crepe bandages
- an eye bath
- antiseptic fluid or cream
- calamine lotion
- an up-to-date first aid reference book
- assorted non-adherent dressings
- paracetamol tablets

Your first aid box is an essential way of keeping useful items together for emergency use. It may be required in a hurry so it must be easily accessible, somewhere where all the staff know and preferably fixed. The container should be clean, dry and airtight. A bathroom is not the ideal place to store the box. Some boxes are locked, but this could pose problems in an emergency if the key is misplaced. It should be clearly labelled and out of the reach of children.

Emotional support of the casualty

As important as the physical needs of the casualty are the psychological or emotional needs. You may only be with your casualty for a short time but during this time you need to build up an element of trust. It is a basic human need to be recognised as an individual, to be valued and to be treated courteously, with dignity and as much privacy as can be afforded at any given time.

Talk to your client, tell him who you are and explain what you are doing to him. This applies even to the unconscious person, as he may still be able to hear you. This helps to allay any fears he may have.

Listen to your client, he may be able to inform you more fully than a witness how the incident occurred. Be aware of any requests made: the client might tell you who to contact about the incident or ask for some medication. It may be a request to pick up a child from school or the nursery. Perhaps he had a pet who ran away after the accident. Any worries or fears your victim suffers will delay recovery and add to the pain he might be experiencing. Reassure him that you will do all you can to help with the request.

People who have attempted to take their own lives need as much, if not more, support as any other casualty.

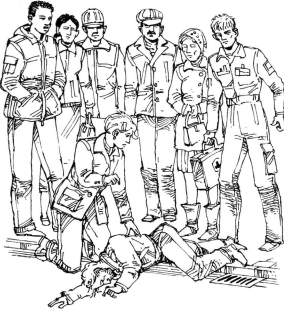

Figure 1.14   *Would you know what to do in an emergency?*

You should act with confidence, as people will quickly become aware of your fears or any lack of confidence. Children are very perceptive. Treating an injured child may require more patience and trust building. Although you should appear confident, always be honest and admit the fact that you might not know what is wrong with the client.

Try not to separate the client, especially the child, from the person he may have been with; to see a familiar face will help him relax more easily. At the same time, maintain privacy if requested, especially from the general public. Allow the client to remain dignified by keeping him covered as much as possible. Treat him as an individual person, not simply a 'casualty'.

Perhaps above all, if you think your victim is seriously ill or dying, do not leave him. Continue to gently talk to him, hold his hand just to let him know that you are there and he is not alone.

Activity 22

Discuss what emotions you think you might experience if you had to deal with somebody who intended taking their own life.

How might these emotions affect the way you treat your clients?

What level of emotional support would you, personally, be able to offer?

BASIC LIFE SAVING TECHNIQUES

Asphyxiation

Scenario

You are one of the carers at a residential home. While on duty during a meal time, suddenly one of your clients begins to cough and choke on her food. She tries to attract your attention. The other residents, alarmed, call for you to help.

COMMENT

ⓘ How would you deal with this situation? In any emergency situation you should act speedily with calmness and efficiency.

Based on what you see and hear, you realise that you need to clear the obstruction from her airway quickly and ensure that your client can breathe as this situation could be life-threatening.

In any emergency situation bear in mind the principles of first aid:

1 Remain calm, think quickly.
2 Do not place yourself in danger.
3 Do not attempt the impossible alone.
4 Quickly assess the situation.
5 Ensure the area is safe.
6 Provide emergency aid.
7 Summon help.

In this situation you would need to act without further upsetting other residents. Clear the area, asking active residents to move – perhaps one may be fit enough to fetch help.

Act quickly, as your client could die if left untreated. She may attempt to breathe but the harder she tries the more firmly lodged the obstruction becomes. Try bending her forward on her chair, so that her head is lower than her chest, slap her up to five times sharply between the shoulder blades, to see if she is able to cough out the food. If this method does not work attempt the abdominal thrust.

THE HEIMLICH MANOEUVRE

The abdominal thrust, or Heimlich manoeuvre, should only be used on adults, not children and young babies.

Providing your client is conscious you can perform this manoeuvre with her sitting or standing. Stand behind her, put your arms round her waist and make a fist with one hand. Place your thumb side slightly above her navel and well below her ribcage. Holding your fist with your other hand, give three or four quick, strong pulls diagonally upwards, towards you. Use your hands to create pressure, do not just squeeze with your arms. Once food is dislodged and coughed from your client's throat, reassure her, let her rest and report the incident to the person in charge. Encourage others to resume eating. Go back to your client and make sure she is not too upset by the incident.

Activity 23

📖❓ Discuss in small groups how you might feel after dealing with a situation like this. What support would you expect from other staff? Discuss what problems you might encounter if dealing with such an emergency situation. Would it be a good idea to determine why your client was choking in the first place?

COMMENT

ⓘ After coping with a choking episode you may feel in shock, or perhaps surprised and pleased that you coped well. Afterwards, you may expect extra consideration from colleagues and might seek to take precautions in case of similar episodes in the future, e.g. checking client's dentures fit correctly and briefing all clients to stay calm.

If a client is unconscious and choking you should apply the Heimlich manoeuvre with him on his back. Safely lower him to the floor, preferably with help, taking care not to strain or injure your back. Kneel astride his hips, placing your hand just above his navel. Push on it with your other hand, thrust at an angle downwards towards his head. Clear food, or other objects, from his mouth so that he does not choke again. Take care not to push food back down the throat. Place him in the recovery position and seek medical aid.

Choking also easily occurs in infants and children. You may need to dislodge foreign bodies (e.g. peanuts are a common cause of choking in youngsters). Place the child over your knee with her head hanging down and apply several slaps between their shoulder blades. Gravity may help to dislodge any obstruction. Once the obstruction is dislodged, reassure and help the child by not leaving her. Seek medical advice. Resuscitation of a child should be taught by people trained to teach first aid.

ARTIFICIAL RESPIRATION

Before carrying out any resuscitation you should have regular practical training.

If your choking client begins to asphyxiate (suffocate) and loses full consciousness, you need to act quickly to save his life.

- Once the obstruction is cleared, check if breathing has stopped. Listen near the nose or mouth, and look for movement of the chest wall. Hold a mirror or shiny object near the mouth to check for condensation.
- If you are sure the client is not breathing, quickly lay him on his back and remove any obstructions from his mouth – e.g. false teeth, blood or vomit. Loosen tight clothing around his neck and tilt his head backwards, lifting the jaw. This opens up the windpipe, or trachea, and keeps the tongue clear.
- Pinch his nostrils together and breathe into the open mouth, or keep the mouth firmly closed and breathe into the nose – with a small child breathe into mouth and nose simultaneously. Some people have a tracheotomy and in this case you would

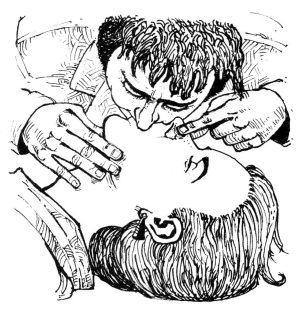

Figure 1.15   *Artificial respiration*

have to check the hole in their neck for obstructions, and breathe into this.

- Blow steadily until the chest wall rises. Remove your mouth, allowing the chest to deflate, and repeat quickly twice to supply oxygen to the blood. Then maintain a steady pace, blowing once every five seconds.
- Ensure that the head is tilted well back and you have a good seal over the mouth.
- If the client vomits, turn his head gently to one side, clear his mouth and throat and then continue artificial respiration until he can breathe for himself. Then place the client in the recovery position, and watch him carefully until help arrives.
- If breathing stops you would need to restart resuscitation. Ensure the heart is still beating, listen against the chest wall. Feel for pulses at the wrist, or the carotid pulse at the side of the Adam's Apple in the neck.

Activity 24

Consider similar situations which might arise, or have occurred, in your work environment. Think about and note down how you would react in these situations. How would you know if your actions had been successful? Consider how the client might feel during and after a choking experience and what reassurance they might need.

Cardiopulmonary resuscitation

If the heart should stop, you need to lay your client flat on her back, taking care not to injure yourself or further injure her.

- Place the heel of one hand over the centre lower part of the breastbone (one finger's breadth below a line joining the nipples) and place the heel of the other on top.
- Keeping your palms and fingers raised

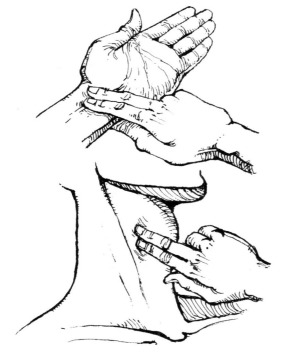

Figure 1.16   *Neck and wrist pulse points*

with straight arms, rock backwards and forwards.
- After each fifth compression blow deeply into the airway.
- If alone, make fifteen compressions to two lung inflations.
- Check the client's pulses every minute, then every three minutes, and continue until medical help arrives or your client becomes conscious, then reassure her and stay with her. This is cardiopulmonary resuscitation (CPR). If she stops breathing the heart may still beat – but if the heart stops beating, breathing will cease.

Resuscitation of a baby or child should be taught to you by somebody trained to teach first aid.

Activity 25

In groups of three practice CPR. You need to obtain access to a resuscitation doll (Recus Annie). Take turns resuscitating it on your own, then with two people, leaving one person as an observer. On one of the more expensive models you are able to check if you were successfully able to resuscitate the doll as lights come on when your technique maintains adequate lung inflation and circulation.

The recovery position

1 Turn the client's head towards you and tilt it back to open the airway.
2 Put the client's arm by their side and, placing their other arm across their chest, bend their far leg under the knee or ankle.
3 Support their head and pull them towards you, on to their side.
4 Support their body against your knees, positioning their head so the airway is open.
5 Bend their upper leg.
6 Put their arm in place to prevent them rolling.

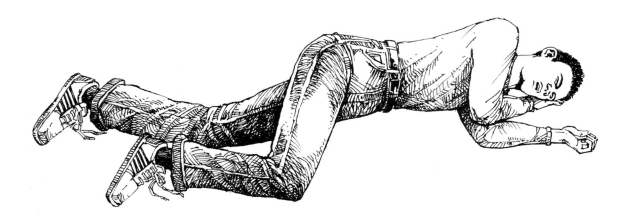

Figure 1.17   *The recovery position*

Activity 26

 In groups of three take it in turns to be an unconscious client, a person administering aid and an observer. Practice in turn putting a client into the recovery position. It is the job of the observer to ensure that he or she is positioned correctly and safely.

COMMENT

ⓘ Why do we need to use this position?

1 To maintain an open airway

2 To allow vomit to drain from client's mouth and prevent choking

There may be times when the recovery position is impossible due to fractures (broken bones) of the back, or neck or head injuries. (First Aid lectures would show you how to deal with all emergency situations correctly – take advantage of any available locally.)

While helping your client, offer constant reassurance and keep them calm. Do not allow them to eat or drink, especially alcohol. Check, recording if possible, the client's breathing and pulse rate per minute, and assess whether your client is awake, drowsy or unrousable – their level of consciousness. Resuscitate the client if necessary. When professional help arrives, give all the available information to the doctor or ambulance team who will take over.

It is important to recognise your limitations. If you are unsure what you are capable of, concentrate on what you know and await help. You are not a doctor or trained nurse and are not expected to act like one.

Haemorrhage

Haemorrhage may be a simple cut or more serious bleeding. Bleeding can be internal or external. Internal bleeding may be worse as it may result from a fracture and is not easy to detect. Reassure your client, keep him warm and comfortable, while waiting for help. Treat external bleeding promptly by applying pressure directly to the wound with a pad of clean material, if available. If a foreign body is present apply pressure to the side of it. To treat an injured limb, support the limb in a raised position as this reduces the pressure of blood flowing into the wound. However, do not attempt to do this unless you are certain that there are no fractured (broken) or dislocated bones. Apply pressure to the wound for about 10 minutes. If the blood has started to clot, cover the area with a sterile or clean dressing and secure the dressing firmly.

Clean minor cuts or abrasions with running water, dry and cover them with a plaster or non-adherent material. Spurting bright red blood comes from an artery and is very serious, so treat it as a priority.

Shock

Shock may be the result of:

- heavy blood loss
- heavy loss of other body fluids, e.g. diarrhoea, vomiting or burns
- accident or injury
- sudden illness
- pain
- heart attack or coronary thrombosis

It is brought about by a reduced blood supply and therefore reduced oxygen to the brain and other organs. Typical signs include:

- pale/greyish colour
- cold clammy skin
- feeling weak, faint, giddy
- blurred vision, nausea, vomiting
- weak, rapid pulse
- shallow, fast breathing
- restlessness, anxiousness, which may progress to unconsciousness

Reassure your client without moving her unnecessarily, stay with her until trained help arrives and she has been transferred to hospital. Lay her down, keeping her head low to one side to reduce the danger of vomiting, and loosen tight clothing. If you are sure there are no broken bones raise both legs to increase the blood supply to the brain. Lightly cover her with a blanket, if available. Do not offer anything to eat, drink or smoke, although you might moisten her lips. Treat any obvious cause of shock, e.g. bleeding. Check the client's breathing, pulse rate and level of consciousness every 10 minutes. If breathing deteriorates or the client vomits, place her in the recovery position and perform CPR if necessary. As soon as possible arrange a transfer to hospital.

SUMMARY

- Deal with emergency situations by relevant action administered promptly, calmly and efficiently.
- When administering emergency aid attempt to preserve life, limit the effects of the condition and promote recovery. Do not delay in summoning help.
- If responding to a health emergency ensure you are not placing yourself in any danger.
- Remember the A, B, C of resuscitation – airway, breathing, circulation.
- Ensure a safe working environment. You

have a responsibility to yourself, colleagues and clients.

- Look towards prevention of accidents but be aware of how to contact the GP and emergency services nearby.
- Accept your limitations and recognise when to ask for the help of carers and colleagues and when to call a GP or the emergency services.
- Maintain your own safety and protection from infection or injury.
- Stick to the policies and protocols (Universal Precautions, the Health and Safety Act (1974) and local policies) – they are there for your own and for others safety.
- Use the correct equipment provided/available.
- Maintain a high level of communication. Always report back to the person in charge.

2

INFLUENCES ON HEALTH AND WELL-BEING

AIMS AND OBJECTIVES

This chapter aims to help students understand health and well-being by considering personal development, inter-personal relationships and relationships within society.

By the end of this chapter you should be able to:

• explain the main characteristics of development in different life stages

• describe ways in which individuals manage change

• describe relationships formed in the contexts of daily life

• investigate the interaction of individuals within society

• compare the characteristics of different social and economic groups

---

The development of individuals: how they manage change

When we are young, it is difficult to look forward and imagine what it will be like to be old, disabled or dependent. On the other hand, think back to when you were a young child: can you remember what it was like to be surrounded by a land of giants? If you visited a strange place or a different country, then you would probably be anxious, confused or scared by your surroundings.

Life is rather like this, a whole series of new situations and challenges, called *life stages*: we move from surroundings where we are comfortable into new and strange ones. From the very beginning, when birth propels the baby from a comfortable, well protected environment into a world where everything is so loud and unfamiliar, we have to learn to cope with each change as it comes along.

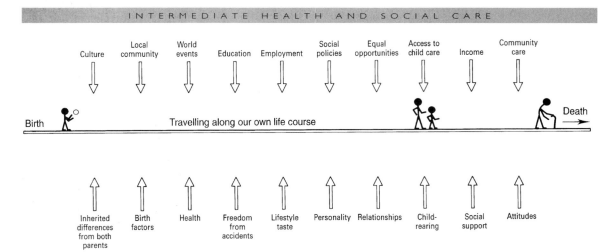

Figure 2.1   *We all go through different life-stages*

Activity 1

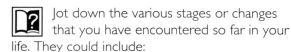 Jot down the various stages or changes that you have encountered so far in your life. They could include:

- learning to walk
- starting school
- changing school
- teenage years
- your first boy or girlfriend.

Now jot down the stages you think you may go through during the rest of your life.

COMMENT

Perhaps you have listed leaving school or college, getting a job and your first pay packet, leaving home to live with friends or in your own flat, getting married, having a child. Few of us like to think further forward than that. It is, we hope, a long time before having to think of the children growing up and leaving home, our own working life coming to an end, and of old age creeping nearer.

This section looks at how we all grow and develop throughout our life, and how our body and mind allow us to adjust and cope with the various situations we face. Look at the list of definitions on page 61 to make sure you understand the terms used in this chapter.

LIFE STAGES

Pre-birth

From the moment of conception, when the female egg is fertilised by the male sperm, many of the characteristics we are born with are already determined for us. Things like the colour of the hair, eyes, skin, shape of face, nose, size, height, and even long-term health are given by the mother and the father when the egg and the sperm, containing the genes, join to form one cell; the male genes decide what sex the baby will be. Some of these inherited characteristics can be influenced by lifestyle, especially eating habits, exercise and smoking, during both pregnancy and future life.

Birth and early years

A human baby needs a lot of care and support, but as soon as it is born, the baby is able to breathe, cry, suck, communicate and get rid of its waste products. It has a number of reflexes, automatic actions, that it needs to survive; for example:

- the 'rooting' reflex, where the baby will turn its head when touched on the cheek
- it searches with its mouth and starts sucking on anything
- the baby is able to move its limbs.

Much of the child's time is spent sleeping, only waking to be fed and changed. The baby can differentiate between stationary black and white and solid grey. Hearing has developed well before birth, and the baby can distinguish its mother's voice. New babies show a dislike of sour tastes, but they recognise the smell of mother's milk.

Over the next few weeks and months the baby develops quickly, gaining many new skills. Do remember that the ages stated are only the *norm*, and that some babies will reach a particular *milestone* earlier, while many will take a lot longer.

Activity 2

1 In pairs, re-read the definitions of growth, development, norm and milestones.

2 Make a list of the various milestones a baby achieves in the first three years, such as smiling, crawling, walking, cutting first teeth. Then decide how old the baby will be at each stage.

3 Compare your list with a friend and see how different they are. Try to come to some agreement.

4 Now check your combined list with Table 2.1 on page 50 and see how accurate you were.

5 If there are any stages not on the chart, find a book on child growth and development and look them up.

COMMENT

Did you find that there were any stages where the age you said was very different from the norm? If so, was it just a guess or were you basing your judgement on a child you know? Perhaps the child you know is more advanced in some aspects. Are there other areas where perhaps he or she is not quite so advanced? This is quite normal.

You should have identified that a child will crawl at about 8 months, walk unaided at approximately 15 months, and will use a small number of words at a year.

Activity 3

After studying Table 2.1, visit a playgroup, nursery school or toddler group. Watch a number of children over a short period of time. Watch what they are doing and try to estimate their age. Find out how old they are and compare it with your estimate.

COMMENT

What were the key activities that helped you identify the ages of the children? Did you base your decision on things like the language the child used? The ability to perform certain tasks or skills in walking, running, etc.?

A child holding an object such as a crayon, between the fingers, rather than just as a fist, will be at least two years old. If a child is rather unsteady walking and easily overbalances, then he or she is probably under 15 months.

Try this activity again at a later time and see if your estimates are better this time.

Cognitive development

The young child does not only develop physically, but also socially and mentally.

Table 2.1 Different stages of childhood development, from birth to two years

Approx. age	1 mth	3 mths	5 mths	8 mths	12 mths	15 mths	18–24 mths
Movement, rest and co-ordination	Exercises legs and arms. Grips with hands. Sleeps for long periods. Sucks, turns opening mouth when touched on cheek.	Explores own hands, fingers, toes and ears. Sleeps 18–20 hours. Begins to take solids. Recognises tastes.	Examines surroundings. Attempts to sit up alone, rolls over and clings to things, furniture and toys. Puts everything into mouth. Co-ordinates movements. Sleeps 10–20 hours.	Sits alone. May crawl, shuffles along, not sure of balance. Examines everything, puts it in mouth and chews. Sleeps 10–16 hours. Active arms and legs. Handles toys and objects.	Curious about everything in reach. Walks around furniture. Stands alone. Uses both hands freely. Able to use finger and thumb grip. Indicates where toys are.	Walks, still unsteady. Picks up small objects. Builds with bricks. Explores everything everywhere.	Walks and runs. Can go up and down stairs by self. Picks up small things. Takes off shoes and socks. Drinks without spilling.
Language and communicating	Crys when hungry or uncomfortable. Grunts and sneezes. Startled by loud noises.	Cries, babbles, laughs, reacts to sounds and movements. Recognises mother quickly, less sure of others.	Cries when wet, dirty, hungry, in pain or when voices raised in anger. Shouts and screams.	Frustrated if unable to have wants satisfied. Needs cuddling when feels unsure. Dribbles, laughs. Vocalises and copies sounds. Attention held for one minute. Teething. Distinguishes between parents and others.	Demonstrates affection and wants cuddling at any time. Likes company and interest. Recognises tones in voices – anger, disapproval and pleasure. Responds well to simple demands. Can use a small number of words – especially 'No'.	Speech – jabbers loudly, uses a range of words. Begins to have temper tantrums. Asserts willpower. Great need for adults' reassurance. Needs cuddle and kiss to comfort.	Puts words together. Copies adult activities, enacting domestic routines. Love/hate relationship. Likes affection, demands attention. Tantrum when frustrated, but easily distracted. Will play alone but prefers to be within hearing of parent. Repeats adult words, copying parrot fashion.

Stimulation using all the senses is an essential part of this process. From birth the baby gains information from its surroundings, how it is handled, what it touches and how it is talked to. As we can see from Table 2.1, by the age of five months a baby can recognise and will be frightened by voices raised in anger. Even a small baby reacts to loud sounds.

Intelligence or cognitive ability is partly inherited, being passed down in the parents' genes, but it is also influenced by the amount of stimulation the developing child is given, as well as by getting adequate nutrition while growing.

Talking to a baby or young child every time you do anything to it, hold it or while it is awake, encourages it to take an interest, to build up a good relationship or bond, and helps it learn a wider range of words. Think how easily we all pick up our own language, but trying to learn a foreign language at school is much harder. That is because it is not being used all around us. Because they are surrounded by a language, children learn words almost without meaning to. Children who are taught two languages right from the beginning can switch from one to another with no difficulty, and are not any more intelligent than those who only speak one.

Social development

Communications are not limited to talking. The child gains information through watching its mother's face, checking for approval and that she does not see anything wrong in what is happening around her.

Play is the way a young child learns. There are six stages of play:

1 solo play – at first, play is led by the parent, or is by oneself
2 onlooking play – as the child begins to mix, he or she gradually realises that others are playing, and may watch them
3 parallel play – children start to play in the company of others, using the same toys, but each playing in their own way
4 joining in play – the play begins to overlap between children
5 simple co-operative play – they find that they can have more fun by sharing toys and equipment
6 complex co-operative play – children develop and act out real life situations: doctors and nurses, school and teacher, mums and dads.

Play enables the child to practice and perfect skills they have seen or been taught. They use it to make sense of their world and to act out everyday events and situations. It also helps them to increase their circle of friends, enabling them to mix and communicate with others. It is important, especially for an only child, to mix with others by joining a playgroup or mother and toddler group. Otherwise, as an adult they will find it difficult to mix and make friends with others.

Activity 4

Watch children at play. How many of the different types of play you can see? Note down examples when play encourages the children to communicate. See if you can identify when the children are 'acting out' everyday situations.

Discuss in your group what skills you identified the children developing and give examples. They might be *social* skills – communication, interacting with others; *physical* skills, such as manual dexterity – drawing, cutting, balancing and placing bricks; or *intellectual* skills like counting, matching shapes in jigsaw puzzles and recognising colours.

Are there other activities they could do to practise the same skills? Do they develop more than one skill within the same play activity?

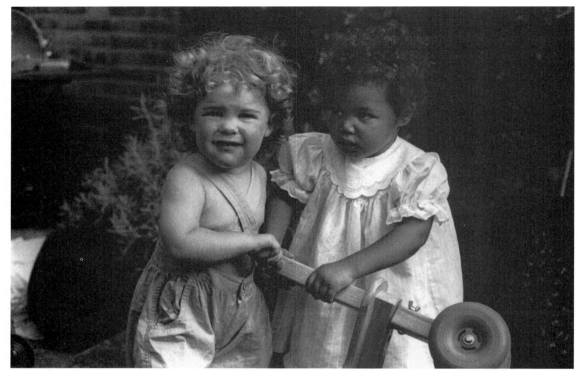

Figure 2.2   *Learning to share is not always easy*

COMMENT

ⓘ Cutting out shapes not only develops the co-ordination needed to use scissors, but it also involves recognising the shapes and may develop language skills as the different ones are identified.

Drawing is not just about holding the crayon; it teaches the difference between colours and shapes, and develops language and communication as the child describes what they have drawn. Additionally it can involve copying shapes, as a pre-reading exercise or learning the co-ordination and visual skills required to colour between lines.

School age

This is a very big step for any child. Suddenly they are separated from their parents for a long period of time and have to compete for the attention of perhaps one adult against a large number of other children. They usually settle down quickly to the routine, choosing friends and developing an understanding of the rules. They are naturally competitive, arguing over who can run the fastest, who has the biggest house, car or any other belonging. The mutual exploration of the body which begins at two or three years, changes to awareness and they become very self-conscious, hiding from others when it is time to change for games or other activities. Their imagination develops, and affects their type of play. This is the time when imaginary friends can appear and become a very real part of their life. They may also develop fears or worries, which seem irrational to adults but to them are very real and plausible. These often occur through misunderstanding an overheard conversation or event. Right and wrong becomes meaningful at this age, and they have an acute and very logical sense of fairness. The idea of timing is slowly understood, initially just past, present and an anticipation of the future, but by eight or nine years they can understand the concept of 24 hours in the day. The family is of great importance. Children act out or re-tell family situations with great detail and accuracy. But at this age they are very ego-centric – self is all important, and in drawings they will often depict themselves as much larger than all those around them.

Pre-teen child

The hand/eye co-ordination is well developed, enabling the child to acquire sophisti-cated reading, writing and drawing skills, easily manipulating hand held computer games. They can pick up computer skills, working videos and other equipment by trial and error without referring to instruction manuals. Games become very intricate, with lots of rules and structure which are often incomprehensible to adults or outsiders. These can be dropped and picked up again whenever time allows, just continuing from where they were left off. While, at this age, children are very competitive, they like to belong to and develop gangs or groups. They frequently make one or two lifelong friendships, and will have a best mate or best friend, usually of the same sex. These friendships can help make the change of school, which often occurs at this time, less traumatic, but if the friends do not go to the same school it can have a long lasting effect.

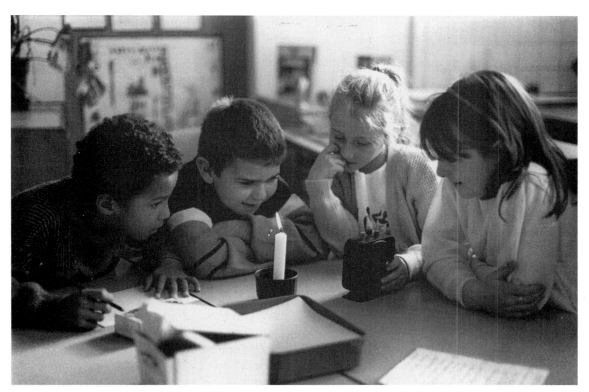

Figure 2.3   *Do you remember your early years in school?*

Reasoning is very matter of fact and logical to the extreme. Things either work or they don't. Given a problem they can gradually work out a solution, but they need some prompting.

Teenage years

A time of great change and turbulence, both in physical development and in relationships with family, friends and within oneself. Although this is a period when they develop their own self identity, and start to take control in decision making, it is also a time when peer pressure and the desire to conform is at its greatest.

Physically there is a huge growth spurt, of approximately 23–46 cms (9–18 ins), over a period of eighteen months to three years. This occurs in girls roughly a year before boys and heralds sexual development. As the hormone levels fluctuate to control this, mood swings occur. Relationships are explored, both emotional and sexual. Secondary sex characteristics (formation of breasts, changes to the scrotum, body and facial hair) are developed along with changes to the general body shape.

Intellectually they develop abstract reasoning, seeing the relationship between concepts and using simple lateral thinking. They tend to be very moralistic, and still very idealistic. Life is very much black or white, with few or no grey areas. At this age the teenager is very aware of right and wrong, but many choose to break the rules, frequently through peer pressure or the influence of an older person.

Appearance is all-important, either to conform to the group's norms or used as a shock tactic. They swing between paying minute attention to detail, to showing total disregard. This often relates to aspects of the same issue, like hygiene or clothes, and seems very confusing to all, the teenager and parents.

It is a time to appear to rebel against the establishment and authority, testing the boundaries to the limit. Although they appear not to value the family, underneath is a desperate desire to be loved and cared for; but they do test that love to the extreme.

While their whole life seems to be in total turmoil, they are also trying to make long-term plans for their future. At school they are having to make choices about which subjects they want to take and those to drop, all at a time when the last thing they want to take is their parents' advice. Work experience during school-time can sometimes help form ideas, but this is often undertaken after the choices have been made. Teenagers who have long-term health problems or illnesses, often use them as another way of gaining some control, sometimes choosing to withhold or delay taking their medication, causing themselves, and their parents, unnecessary suffering and discomfort. Many youngsters at this age may be acting as carers, caring for other children in the family or even for an ill or disabled parent.

Activity 5

In a group, think about and discuss your experience as a teenager. Can you think of times when you thought more of what your friends said than you did of your parents?

How many times have you said, 'I will not do that to a child of mine?' or 'I will let them stay out, go to . . . will let them wear . . .', etc.

In a role-play, think about how you would get permission to go to a party, to stay out with a friend, or what happened when Mum or Dad did not like your new clothes or hairdo. What communication skills did you use? Were they confrontational, or negotiation? Perhaps they were even manipulative, as you tried to play one parent off against the other?

How clear a vision have you for your future? Write it down and look at it again in the future; see how different your life has turned out to be.

Adult life

As we move into adulthood, our life seems to go through yet another period of change. You leave school and no matter how much you have looked forward to that day, there is a certain amount of sadness. The structure for the days is different, with no long summer holiday and regular breaks from school to look forward to. You have to get your first full time job, putting your foot onto the employment ladder. It is very easy to have unrealistic expectations for the future. From being in the senior forms at school, suddenly you become the junior again, having to learn new rules and perhaps new skills in order to do the job. Some people go on to college or university and delay that major move. But there are still important decisions to make, such as which one to go to and where to live. Unfortunately, some do not manage to find employment and this brings its own problems. They should make use of all the agencies available to help the search, instead of just sitting around getting bored.

The school group of friends and peer groups, will probably be swapped for the company of work colleagues, membership of social clubs or linked to a particular hobby. Relationships become closer and the circle of family, friends and regular companions becomes smaller. Major changes may include:

- moving away from the parental home, to share accommodation or to set up one's own home, through renting or buying
- entering a permanent relationship, resulting in marriage and then a family unit.

All of these changes will involve making decisions, sometimes by oneself and sometimes with other people. The financial implications of such changes have a great effect on lifestyle and may influence the choices made.

As experience is gained at work, job opportunities often arise perhaps within the same firm, company, or from outside. These career moves can involve moving away from the immediate area, very different responsibilities or even changes in the hours of work. Career changes seem to occur when the demands at home, of a partner and a young family are at their highest.

The job market has changed greatly over the last decade. Many women with children have now continued with their jobs after maternity leave, or have found part-time employment. This involves finding child care facilities. Grandparents or other members of the family will sometimes provide cover, or working hours may be arranged at weekends or at times when the child's father is home. For both partners, husband and wife, balanc-

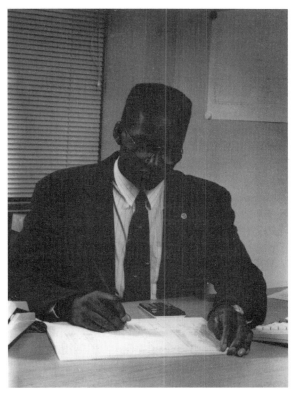

Figure 2.4   *The world of work brings new pressures and responsibilities*

ing the demands of a job, a home and a young family is very difficult and takes a lot of management. Finances are often strained at this time and this can lead to rows and arguments.

Middle life

Slowly but surely the family grows up: parents are confronted by these 'children' who are one day charming and very good company, but who, the next minute, turn into argumentative and unreasonable beings. Although all parents look forward to the time when their children grow up, it still comes as something of a surprise and shock. It may trigger off a period of re-evaluation of life. Certainly it is a time of taking stock. Many people have reached a point at work when they are in positions of responsibility. Others may have reached a stage when they feel frustrated, that opportunities at work, and perhaps at home, have passed them by. The menopause, when a woman's monthly periods cease, indicates the end of being able to have children. Many women see this as a major crisis time. Care needs to be taken over general health, nutrition and fitness to ensure that problems do not occur in the future. Pressures can build up at work and, with difficulties at home, might lead to a general feeling of low self-esteem. Elderly parents often die during this period of life, raising a feeling of vulnerability. This is also a time when a work colleague or friend may suffer an early heart attack. Of course, not everyone is financially secure after a lifetime of work, due to unemployment, short-term contracts and redundancies. All these external influences can cause friction within the marriage, increasing the likelihood of divorce.

On the other hand, it can be a very positive episode when life and its horizons expand. The children are more independent and generally need less supervision, although they can be replaced by elderly, dependant parents. Frequently there are increasing opportunities for holidays, breaks and social opportunities without the children, as they choose to go with friends or remain at home. Relationships are often strong as couples have learnt to work through their problems together. Many take advantage of the opportunity to improve their education by taking further courses, aiding their work options, for leisure pursuits or simply for their own satisfaction. Financially the family is more secure, with outgoings diminishing as mortgage or rent payments level out, and even decreasing while earnings often increase in line with experience. Expenditure on household goods is limited to replacing existing items, rather than trying to furnish from scratch. Children tend to forget this when they leave home, and want to have all the benefits of household appliances and other things that their parents have, instead of having to start with limited belongings.

Separation at this time, through death or divorce, is exceptionally traumatic. The lone partner is left at a time when they might still have many of the family and financial commitments but lessening support networks to draw on. After many years within a partnership, most of their friends and social groups consist of couples and there are difficulties adjusting to life as a single person. Over the years, responsibility for certain 'jobs' will have been delegated, such as the family accounts, gardening, home maintenance, driving or ironing. It takes a long time to sort out how to resume control.

Activity 6

 Talk to a person of your parent's age, but perhaps not your parents. Ask them about their current worries, concerns for their family, job, future or health. How do they view their old age?

Perhaps they identified worries about their parents or their children's future.

They may be concerned about the financial situation, with the children getting older or the home they live in needing repairs.

Later adulthood

Life has changed dramatically for large sections of this age group. Many are no longer existing solely on state pensions, but also have private ones from their work. Improved medical intervention has brought better overall health status, together with a longer life expectancy. Freedom from work and family ties gives them the chance to live life to the full. Others feel consigned to the scrap heap, having been forced to leave work while they still have much to offer.

There is great diversity among older people in retirement, in terms of their financial resources, experiences, expectations, dreams and interests. Adjusting to a lifestyle without work takes effort by all involved. Previous 'demarcation' of jobs needs to be re-thought and role changes negotiated. Hobbies can help give purpose, interest and time for self. But for some who have poured everything into work, this is initially difficult. Many voluntary organisations are grateful to harness the expertise and experience of retired volunteers.

Health changes might be experienced to which the individual or the environment needs to adapt. For example, changes in eyesight require the use of glasses, but perhaps will also benefit from improved lighting in and around the home. Local services may need to be utilised to enable people to maintain their independence at home. Choosing to move to more suitable housing is a major decision, often faced when a partner dies. This makes it all the more poignant, as

memories are tied up with the home. There are now many alternative forms of accommodation from residential homes through to mini villages, that provide the freedom of living independently with the protection and back-up of services and a warden on site. The maintenance of a large family home can be a problem financially, physically and for the immediate family.

However, old age can be a positive and rewarding time of life, enjoying a new stage of life's journey while reflecting on what has been experienced: see Fig. 4.5. As the individual grows and develops to maturity many crisis periods are negotiated. There are many circumstances that influence the choices that need to be made at each point: family, culture, religion and job prospects are just some of them. Most people live a healthy and reasonably happy life, although perhaps we all carry dreams of what might have been.

COPING WITH LIFE'S CHANGES

As we have seen, there are a number of events that occur during one's lifetime which will cause major changes to lifestyle. As we pass through different life stages, some changes can be anticipated, but others may not happen to everyone, or may not occur at a definite time of life: they are unpredictable. How we learn to react to these changes and the help we receive will affect both our ability to cope and also the health of all those involved.

Activity 7

1 Working in pairs, make two lists: one of predictable life changes and one of unpredictable changes.

2 Jot down next to each one the period of your life in which they are likely to occur.

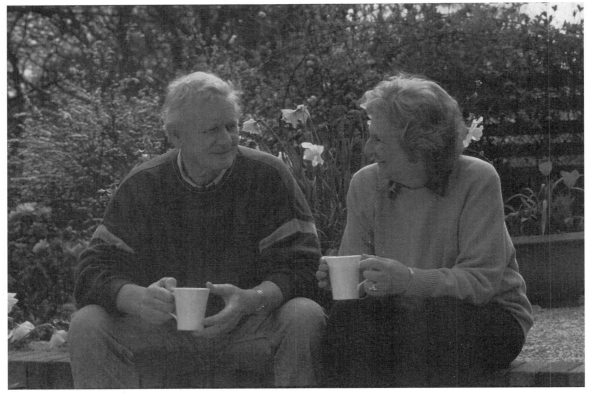

Figure 2.5   *A lifetime companion can bring many joys*

COMMENT

 The list of predictable events might have included:

- starting and leaving school
- getting married
- moving house
- starting work.

Unpredictable changes you might have listed are:

- family separations
- divorce
- redundancy
- serious illness or injury.

Most of these events will occur during set times of your life, but some of them can happen both during childhood and adult life.

Although the timing may be different, many of the ways in which you might cope with these events are similar.

Activity 8

 In groups of 4–6, discuss what help you would need to cope with any of these events.

COMMENT

 This could be developed into a group or personal project. The aim is to find and present in either written or verbal form, information about the various agencies available for help in these circumstances. This information should include how to get help or advice:

- Do you have to be referred to them or can you approach them yourself?

- Is the service free or will it cost?

- Can you use the service as much as you want or are there any limits?

Some of these services or agencies would include:

career advice, estate agents, Citizens Advice Bureau, financial advice and counselling, marriage advice, Relate, solicitors, social services, local church, medical and nursing advice and support, bereavement support, undertakers.

(This is not an exhaustive list. There are many more services, but some may only be available within your immediate area.)

These are the more formal services and agencies that can give help and advice at times of need. However, most people turn initially to members of their own family, or circle of friends. A child is likely to look to his or her parents or peers for immediate help and support, and so might an adult. This informal network is an important forum which allows the person to talk through and generally discuss the wide range of feelings and emotions that are always generated by a major life change.

However, caution must be noted. The fact that these people are family or close friends means that they are unlikely to be able to give an impartial or unbiased point of view. Indeed, if they do so, it might feel as though they are not giving the support the person needs. More importantly, friends and relatives may give inaccurate advice and not be aware of the services and support groups currently available.

Activity 9

 In groups, discuss how coping with one of these changes can affect your health, and what can be done to limit the effects.

COMMENT

- Inability to sleep and lack of appetite are two of the most common symptoms that can in the long term have a dramatic effect of one's health.

- Other problems might include poor communication leading to a breakdown in relationships; disability which can lead to other health problems; coping with disability while causing pain and discomfort in the carer.

- Additional problems include poor personal hygiene due to lack of interest or inability to cope with bathing.

Some of the support network identified above will be among those utilised in coping in these circumstances. Formal counselling and help from various self-help agencies can be an invaluable source of help. Family and friends can be of help, not only by providing a listening ear, but by giving encouragement to seek help and providing much needed relief with things like babysitting, shopping, general chores and other such activities. Many people are reluctant to ask for help, so others may have to offer the support and help.

You have been looking at some of the knock-on effects of life's events and some of the techniques and help that can be drawn on in order to cope with the changes that you will experience. By using this knowledge you will be able to help yourself, family friends and clients in times of need.

SELF CONCEPT

Through this chapter we have been looking at the development of an individual mainly in relationship to age. During childhood we soon develop a concept of *ourself*. Many things contribute to a general feel of self-worth.

Activity 10

- List how people influence the way you feel about yourself.
- Identify those people.

COMMENT

You may have listed things such as how people speak to you, what they call you, whether they are friends or family, a boy-friend or a girl-friend. Do those people pay you compliments? Do they care about you and what you think? Do they say that you have done something well, or thank you for helping them?

A child needs to grow up in a home where those around show that he or she is valued as a person, and that what the child says or does is important; when the child has something to say then someone listens and is interested in the conversation; even small achievements are praised, and the adult shows pride in that achievement. The child is then likely to grow up with a high feeling of self-worth. On the other hand, if the child is always criticised, told that he or she is stupid and any achievement is ridiculed, the child will then grow to feel a failure with low esteem and low self-worth.

There are, frequently, other people who provide the personal interest that everyone needs. These could be a neighbour, a close relative or even a school teacher; someone who shows an interest and cares what the child is doing and achieving. If that interest is not given, it is likely that the child will grow up with very negative feelings about themselves. This could lead to not achieving at school, to truancy and even to getting involved in crime or drugs.

Sometimes a young person who feels un-loved and under-valued may try and fill that void by entering into an intense sexual relationship. This is done in effort to try to obtain a partner who will love and care. A child may be conceived as part of that relationship through the desire to produce a baby, or to create a belonging that will automatically give love. All these alternatives are rather drastic options, that in the long run are more likely to bring further upset and pain.

So by what other means can we try to raise our own self-esteem? Firstly, you have to learn to like yourself and learn to be honest about the things you do. You need to focus not on what you dislike about yourself, but on what you can be proud of.

Activity 11

Jot down the things that you have done in the past two or three days that you can be proud of. They need not be large things, but things that you have done well or achieved, when you thought you might not be able.

COMMENT

These could be all kinds of things, including:

- doing a job for one of the family
- learning some new words in a different language
- completing your homework
- getting a higher grade than normal
- not arguing with your younger brother or sister for an evening
- dressing or changing your appearance so that someone pays you a compliment.

We are not good at giving ourselves a pat on the back, or praising others when we feel they have done well.

Try thanking one of the family for something they have done, or your teachers for the lessons they have just completed. Not only will it make their day, but it will also give you a good feeling about yourself, especially if they respond favourably. Each night, list at least three things you have done during the day, that you feel good about and are proud of achieving. Try to do this on a regular basis; at first you will find it difficult, but as you begin to value yourself more it will become easier.

Activity 12

This activity needs to be co-ordinated and is better conducted within small groups of students who are comfortable with each other.

Take a few pieces of paper, one for each other member of the group. On each piece of paper, write a student's name, and two or three words which you feel describes the positive attributes of that student.

The co-ordinator gathers in the papers and collates the comments. Written or verbal feedback is given to each student, of their attributes identified by the group (this is in order to prevent any personalisation or recognition of handwriting).

COMMENT

The exercise enables you to have feedback on how you appear to others. It can be a useful starting point to build on and develop your positive attributes. The feedback can also be utilised in the preparation of your own Curriculum Vitae (CV).

SUMMARY

- A positive view of oneself allows an individual to grow and cope with life's challenges.

- It also enables the development of meaningful friendships and relationships.

- Life will not always be smooth, but with a high self-esteem even major changes in life can be negotiated and overcome.

DEFINITIONS

Growth The changes in length and size, often measured by height and weight. Some children grow quickly, while others grow more steadily.

Development The complex changes that occur in the function of an individual, like learning to walk, speak, write. It is more difficult to measure and is usually compared with the norm (see below). Just as children grow at different rates, development is similarly affected.

Norm The measurement of an average standard, pattern or stage considered to be representative of a group (in this case, children or adults). When comparing children's ability with what a book says is normal, it is important to remember that some children acquire skills early, while others may take much longer.

Milestones The key stages that a child will achieve during their growth and development. If a child regularly falls behind in reaching these stages, then the doctor or health visitor may be concerned and wish to keep a more regular check.

Genes The inherited characteristics or blueprints passed on to the mother and father at conception. Genes are contained within the nucleus of the sperm and egg.

Cognitive The mental function of the brain: the function and capacity to understand and reason.

Interpersonal relationships: their influence on health and well-being

EVERYDAY RELATIONSHIPS

We are in relationships from the cradle to the grave. During this time we have a number of different relationships, e.g. at work, in our family, with our friends. Some of these relationships are quite formal, and have strict rules. At work our relationship with a manager may be limited to discussion about getting the job done.

It is usually more difficult to relax and laugh with a manager or teacher than your work-mates or fellow students. It is unlikely that you would be able to get away with saying the same sort of things to your friends as you would say to a brother, sister or parent. If, for example, you were angry with your mother, you might start shouting at her or banging things about. If you did that to a friend in a classroom or office, you would probably feel embarrassed and look stupid in the eyes of the others.

Why do different relationships have different 'rules'? Usually, the closer we are to peo-

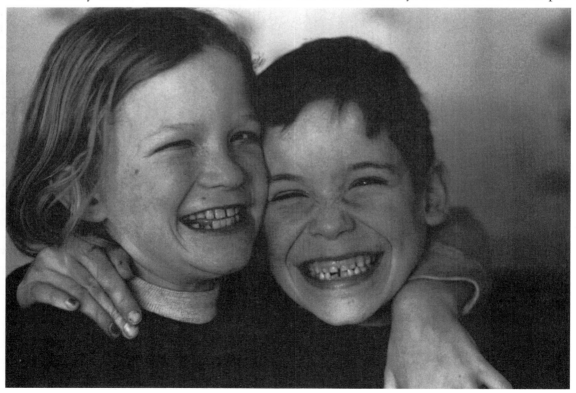

Figure 2.6   *The relationship between brother and sister can have a large effect on family and social life*

ple the less likely it is that a person will reject us. Getting closer to people can be seen as a series of risky steps, each one exposing more of our personality (the good and the bad parts) to the other person. As we become closer we can behave more naturally because we know that they will accept us as we are, and we don't have to put on an act. This process can happen over a long period of time or suddenly, when someone pours their heart out. When people are very close there can be strong feelings of love, anger, jealousy, sexual attraction and even hate. These feelings can get in the way of family life and the smooth running of a class or business, so we use 'rules' – ways of saying what people should and should not do in a given social situation.

CASE STUDY I

Let us see how this idea of 'social rules' could apply in the case of a Saturday for a 16-year-old boy.

Alan wakes up to hear his sister Sue having an argument with his little brother John. He shouts to them to be quiet, but it does not work so he puts his head under the pillow and tries to get back to sleep. Just as he gets back to sleep, having a dream about a girl he likes, his mum comes in and wakes him, telling him that ten o'clock is too late to be in bed and that he promised to take his little brother to a shop. Although he complains, Alan knows he will have to get up now because he does not want an argument and that John has been really looking forward to going into town with him. There is also a chance that the girl he had just been dreaming about might be working at the shop that day. Despite this he argues a bit with his mum just to show he is not a pushover. As it happens his friend is not at the shop as he had hoped, and he is disappointed because he wanted to arrange a meeting later. On the way home he is short-tempered with John, who starts to cry. Alan then feels guilty and worried that he will be told off by his mother again.

For a while Alan is a bit moody and after a few attempts to chat with him, the family leave him alone in his room. A couple of hours later Alan is wondering why the house is so quiet so he looks around to find everyone has gone out (his music

was so loud he did not hear their goodbyes). This makes things worse. No-one seems to understand him today, especially himself. Alan heats a pizza and makes some hot chocolate, which spills over the hob. He leaves it for mum to sort out – why should he care? He begins to feel a bit better and decides to phone one of his mates, Kev, who agrees to meet in town. Alan knows his mum is not happy about their friendship because Kev has been in quite a bit of trouble. This makes the outing even more worthwhile to Alan because somehow his mum seems to be the cause of everything that has gone wrong today, even though he can't explain why.

The two boys meet up with some other friends and watch an '18' film about a bank robbery that goes wrong and everybody except the hero gets killed.

Over a hamburger and chips Kev shows Alan an expensive looking calculator he stole earlier in the day. Alan admires it, but is not really sure about how he feels. Walking home alone Alan sees Linda (the girl he had hoped to meet earlier), on the other side of the road with a boy from school that he hates. By the time he gets home he feels churned up and his mum, who was ready to scold him about the state of the kitchen, gives him a hug which makes him feel a little better. Alan stays in watching videos that night hoping someone will phone him, but nobody does. He goes to bed feeling confused.

Activity 13

After reading through the above account, list the different relationships that Alan was aware of that Saturday. When you have done this, pick out two relationships which you think are very important to Alan at this time.

- Why do you think these relationships are important?
- What does Alan get from these relationships at this time?
- Why is Alan confused?
- What relationships could have been mentioned but are not?
- What is going on for Alan at this time of his life?

COMMENT

ℹ️ In the example above, Alan is in a number of different relationships. Each relationship brings out a different part of him. The relationship with his mother moves from being like a small child needing comfort to that of a tough young man trying to become independent. Towards his brother he is sometimes like a father and then more of a tormentor. His friend Kev makes him feel more like a tough man until Alan starts wondering about his honesty. Part of him is impressed and part of him thinks Kev is rather sad. Linda is the girlfriend he would like to have, but she does not seem interested.

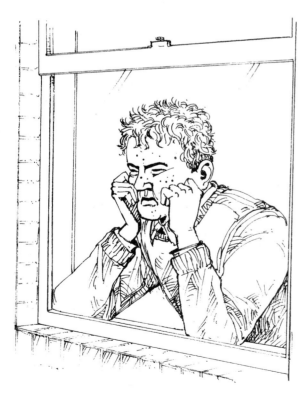

Figure 2.7   *The world can seem a miserable, hostile place for a teenager*

Changes in relationships

We carry lots of different parts of ourselves through all of our lives. In a sense there is a wise old person (perhaps modelled on a grandparent) in a teenager, and a bit of a teenage rebel in some old people who feel pushed around in an elderly persons home. Why is this? At different stages certain needs become more important than others. As babies our primary need is to be loved, fed and cared for. At this stage we are therefore totally dependent. These feelings of dependency can persist and lead us to seek relationships where we are looked after in a way that does not require us to return the care.

As adolescents we become very concerned with identity and therefore experiment with relationships that give us a feeling of what it is like to be in different identities: e.g. raggas, ravers, townies, grungers, etc. In early adulthood most of us become interested in intimate relationships which may lead to stable partnerships and children.

New relationships

All these stages will affect the kind of relationships we have and to some extent we cannot escape the sort of relationships that are a part of the life stage we are in. Quite often people in their mid- to late twenties miss the experience of going out and meeting in groups because all their friends seem to be having children or 'settling down'. We see less of our brothers and sisters as we get older, sometimes with sadness or relief or both. As you could see with Alan, the relationship with a parent can shift from needy child to enemy, to friend, and back again.

Life changes

Sometimes things over which we have little control change our relationships for us.

Where was Alan's father? Perhaps he had left home. This would change the relationship with his mother, and probably brother and sister as well. Maybe Kev will get caught so many times that he will go to prison. Linda might move away. Alan might have a football accident which means that he would not be selected to play for his school. He could then drift away from his football friends and form new friendships somewhere else.

Activity 14

 To find out the effect of changes on relationships you could try this:

Tell your parent or parents that you would like to study the effect of change on their relationship. If they agree, ask the following questions (you could make up a different list if it seems more appropriate):

I   Describe your life and relationships before you became a parent (or parents). What did you do? Where did you go at weekends? What was life like?

2   Now ask the same questions for when they had become parents. Ask how their relationship changed. Did either of them feel left out to make way for the new family member? Did they have less time for each other? How did they get on with in-laws, friends and family? Perhaps one parent left or became ill. Was this a result of becoming a parent or would it have happened anyway?

This activity should show how a major life event such as becoming a parent has a significant effect on virtually all relationships.

WHY DO PEOPLE FORM RELATIONSHIPS?

Professional relationships

Some relationships exist where we have little choice in the matter, such as relationships with employers, teachers, doctors and carers. These are professional relationships which may not offer much chance to get to know a person well. We often have to put up with whatever the person offers, good or bad, because we need the service they are offering more than their interest or companionship. These are relationships we have to make the best of. Sometimes they work well, other times they don't work at all and we have to change jobs or doctors etc. Obviously if we are professionals who are offering a service where we will be forming relationships with clients, patients or residents, then it is important to try to offer the *possibility* of a good working relationship through the use of communication skills.

Social relationships

By social relationships I refer to friends outside the family. These can range from casual acquaintances whom we like, to close friends. They can include friends at work, at a club, in the classroom or the pub. Sometimes we get together to share ideas and find new ways of looking at and thinking about the world around us. These relationships are very important to us, as they provide us with:

• a sense of identity and belonging, knowing who we are, not being lonely.
• a chance to explore different ways of being with people, being funny or serious,

happy and sad.

- finding out about the 'social rules' of a community, knowing what is acceptable or unacceptable and abiding by these rules, or finding people who do not agree with them and challenging them.
- picking up on gossip, learning about ourselves through other people's lives. Seeing someone experience something (like a relationship break-up) may make your own break-up easier to understand and get through (perhaps this is why soap operas are so popular).

Social relationships may develop and become very close, usually when people share parts of themselves they would not want to share with a larger social group.

Close relationships

The more people get to know each other, the closer they get. They may not like what they see but as long as they remain in contact they are close. Letting someone become close to you involves taking risks because they may reject you, so it takes a mixture of courage and need. We all need close relationships as well as social relationships because the parts of us that are not available to social friends are left out. Feelings of vulnerability, strong attraction, love, tenderness and sexual feelings can be kept hidden until we meet someone (e.g. a close friend) with whom we can share these feelings. If we keep these important feelings hidden we run the risk of becoming cut off and perhaps depressed, or being a sort of 'party animal' who never gets close to people and keeps changing friends and partners to avoid getting in touch with feelings they cannot face. Sometimes a counsellor is the first person such an individual might get close to, in order to learn how to be close without falling apart.

THE ROLE OF THE FAMILY IN INDIVIDUAL DEVELOPMENT

CASE STUDY 2

Frank and Sally Turner have been married for 18 years and have three children; Dave aged 17, Paula aged 13 and Sam who is a recent arrival, aged 2. Frank lost his job a year ago and has been spending a lot of time at home between searching for jobs. He is beginning to get quite moody and irritable at times, and sometimes takes it out on the older children. Sally has a part-time job at a nearby school, during which time Frank looks after Sam. Recently Sally's father died after a long illness, and her mother wants to move in with the family. This has produced some bad feeling between Frank and Sally because despite the fact that Sally's mother will bring in a little extra income which is badly needed at this time, Frank resents the idea of her moving in. He has never felt comfortable with her and fears that she might try to take over. His self esteem is not very high at the moment, as nobody seems to want to employ him. He views Sally's mother moving in as the last straw.

Sally and Frank seem to be arguing more these days and Frank has been drinking a lot, which makes matters worse. Dave and Paula are wondering what has happened to their Dad who used to be much more fun than he is now. Sally feels as though she has to hold the family together but gets really tired all the time and worries about her mother. She complains of dizzy spells and headaches which her doctor is unable to find a cause for.

Activity 15

 Discuss the Case Study above, in small groups.

The Turner family seem to be in a dwindling spiral. What is happening to the health and well-being of Frank and Sally, once happily married? How do you think things could end up? Will

Frank and Sally be able to take the strains of staying together or would they be better separating?

Consequences of relationship breakdown on health and well-being

What is happening to family life these days? The idea of the perfect family living in harmony is increasingly seen as an illusion; the image of an extended family shown in Fig. 2.8, in which members support each other is, sadly, not a reality for many people. According to some researchers we are approaching a time when half of all couples will separate before the children are fully grown up. When this happens, the job of parenting is put under great strain and many fathers (for a number of reasons) are unable or unwilling to cope. About 40 per cent of separated fathers lose contact with their children after two years.

Activity 16

 If you can find someone who has been affected by divorce or separation who is willing to talk about it, you could ask the following questions:

How did the separation affect your health and well-being at the time?
Did the separation make a difference to other relationships?
Were your studies or work affected by the separation?
Have there been any long-term effects (e.g. depression) on your health?
Have there been any benefits to you resulting from the separation?

DEPRESSION

Depression is a common result of separation. The sense of loss of a partner to whom someone is close, even if they did not get on well, leaves a black hole which can be difficult to shake off. Everybody gets a bit depressed some of the time, when things go wrong or when we are disappointed. Many of us will get depressed for a while if we lose someone we care for, following bereavement or separation. This will usually lift after a period of grief, or pining for the lost person. Comfort and support at this time are very important. More serious is the kind of depression which goes on for a long time and makes life seem quite pointless. In these cases a health professional such as a doctor or counsellor should be involved.

Being depressed can make everything seem more difficult. It can be hard to get up in the morning, muscles can ache, conversation slows down, people become irritable, moody and tearful. Feeling tired all the time with headaches and loss of appetite is common. A loss of interest in sex and neglect of personal care are also features of depression. In more severe cases suicidal thoughts may be present. Someone who is depressed may drink more or take drugs.

Note: Please do not think that if any of this applies to you then you must be depressed, as these features have to be considered in the *context* of other factors, such as the state of a person's relationships.

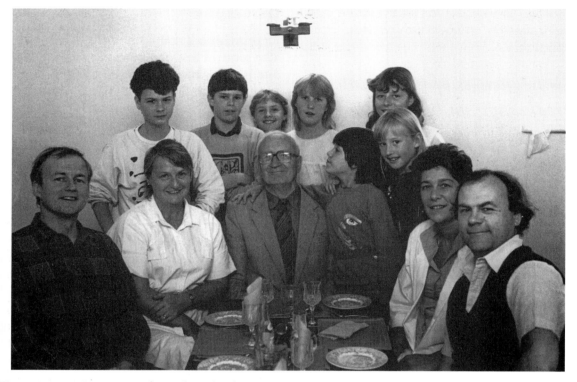

Figure 2.8   *Do you come from a large family?*
Extended families with their support networks are not as common now as in previous generations

The interaction of individuals within society

The aim of this section is to explore the interaction of individuals within society and how they may influence health and well-being. This will include a range of factors such as our own lifestyle as well as social and economic factors.

When you have completed this section you will be able to:

- investigate relationships in society and the different roles adopted by individuals
- describe how laws, rules and social conventions affect the roles of individuals
- compare the characteristics of different social and economic groups using a standard classification system
- identify the possible impact of the characteristics on individual choices which affect health and well-being.

INTRODUCTION

When asked to explain why some people are healthier than others, the usual answer given is that there are biological or natural differences, or some lead a healthier life, i.e. their 'lifestyle' is better than others. It is easier to focus on 'lifestyle' rather than talk about the social factors, such as housing, employment or government policies, which may affect them. We often do this because biological and natural explanations seem to be 'common sense' answers. We need to resort to common sense and experience in order to make sense of, and to function in our everyday lives and the society of which we are a part.

Making sense of society means that we have to make on-the-spot judgements about situations and use our common sense in order to cope. These judgements are often formed by and based on our everyday experiences, and the way in which we were brought up and socialised by our families, schools, churches, clubs and friends. We gradually build up a body of knowledge and experience which helps us explain and understand our lives and our societies. However, our own experiences may be very different from others', as you will discover when you talk to different people.

This section will explore ways in which our behaviour is affected by the roles we play in society and other people's expectations of us in different settings. It will discuss the unwritten rules and social conventions which affect our behaviour, as well as refer to those which are written as Codes of Conduct and laws. This section will also look at how belonging to different social groups may affect our health and well-being. It will enable you to reflect on ideas which you take for granted and provide new insights and ideas for you to examine.

INFLUENCES ON SOCIAL BEHAVIOUR

Let us look at some of the things which affect the way in which we behave. We probably all imagine that we are 'free' agents and

able to make up our minds about what we eat, drink, believe and the ways in which we behave.

Activity 17

Read the following Case Studies and make a list of the ways in which they differ. What are the major influences on their health likely to be?

CASE STUDY 3

Amy is seven years old and she lives with her parents in a three bedroomed house in a residential area of a London borough. Her father is in paid employment in the computer industry and her mother is a nurse in general practice. They are in the proceeds of purchasing the house in which they live. Amy has one older brother who is 15 years old and a 17-year-old sister who is completing her A levels prior to going on to higher education. Her sister wants to be a pharmacist.

The family is English although both sets of grandparents, who also live in London, are from south east Asia. The family are Sikhs and observe the customs and practices which are part of their belief system.

They are non-smokers and do not drink alcohol.

CASE STUDY 4

Joe is the eight-year-old son of Joanna, a single parent living in a rented flat in a multi-tenanted house in London. Joe has a younger sister who is three years old, called Jenni. The children's father visits them and takes them out once a month, but there is no chance of the family living together because of the father's violent outbursts which caused the initial break-up.

Joanna works part-time in the local burger bar while Jenni is cared for by a friend. Joe is taken to school and collected by his mother each day. Joanna works some evenings, when a friend comes to babysit for her. She has a great deal of trouble making ends meet and her income is supported by welfare benefits. The family are Catholic and sometimes attend the local church.

Joanna's parents live in Nottingham and the family meet at major holiday times such as Christmas.

COMMENT

 The differences between the two families are as follows:

- Amy's parents are both in fairly secure employment, which means that there is a regular income. Long-term planning is possible in terms of savings, pension schemes and possibly holidays. As the family is buying their house this will bring a measure of security. This security will probably provide them with sufficient resources in their retirement.

- The families would be categorised as coming from different social classes: i.e. the work that they do is very different. Amy's family would be said to belong to social class 2 and Joe's family to social class 5. You can check the meaning of these social class categories later on in this chapter. (Social class will be discussed in more depth a little later. The social class to which we belong may have long-term implications for our health and well-being.)

- Joe's family is less secure than Amy's family, as his parents are separated and his mother is in part-time employment. This often means that it is difficult to save and plan for the future, there is no access to pension schemes and the mother's income is insufficient to maintain a reasonable lifestyle. This is likely to have adverse effects on resources available during the working life and in retirement. His mother needs welfare benefits to make up her income. Women are more likely than men to be working in part-time employment with low pay.

- There are other differences within each of the families, as each family member may have different aspirations, interests and abilities. They are also of different ages which means that their experiences will be different as new inventions appear on the market, new discoveries are made and new ways of teaching are introduced.

- One example of this is the availability of computing facilities in schools, the home and in the workplace. This may mean that some people are more familiar with and therefore more able to use computers, than others who have not had the same opportunities. Some people may have grown up in a time when there was plenty of employment while others are born and grow up in times of high unemployment and fewer job opportunities. These different experiences play a part in the way we develop both personally and physically.

- The children in both families will be socialised into the beliefs and the traditions of their religions. The cultural factors in both families will also influence their health and social customs.

Both families need good nutrition, safe housing, employment, clothing and the ability to participate in the local community and the society to which they belong. This may mean joining local clubs, participating in school outings and activities, swimming, attending meetings and a whole variety of other ways. The opportunities and resources necessary for such standards may be affected by a number of social and economic factors.

One of the factors which may affect the opportunities and resources for individuals and families is that of social class.

SOCIAL CLASS

Social class is a term used to describe different types of employment, which are grouped together by their similarities to form occupational groups or social classes. Depending upon your occupation you may be assigned to one of these groups which will describe your social class. This administrative system is a shorthand for describing and assigning people to certain groups or categories of people in employment. It is not intended as a way of labelling people, but simply for analysing information from census and other surveys. The most commonly used social class grouping, is that of the Registrar General which falls into five categories:

- Social Class 1 – people who are directors and owners of companies
- Social Class 2 – employed professionals such as teachers, solicitors
- Social Class 3 – non-manual workers such as supervisors, police officers and non-commissioned officers
- Social Class 4 – those who require special skills to undertake the work e.g. carpenter
- Social Class 5 – people in occupations which require little skill

Of course, this list is a simplification of a complex system of analysing people's employment. But you will see that Amy's father's job would be classified as social class 2 and her mother's work would be classified as social class 2 or 3, while Joe's mother's work would be in the social class 5 category.

Income

The social class of an individual is often an indication of their income. The higher up the social scale, the more likely they are to earn more on a regular basis. There are obviously other ways of using the concept of social class but be warned: *it is important that this type of classification does not lead to generalisations about people's lifestyles.* Someone who is a company director may be classified as social class 1, but there are often vast differences in company directorships; one could work for a large company such as ICI or for a small company of two or three employees. Both of these would be social class 1 but each would have vastly different salaries, benefits and lifestyles.

Problems of generalisation

One of the problems with generalisation is that incomplete or incorrect assumptions may be made on a limited basis and associations made between social class and individual behaviour. It is sometimes referred to as 'victim-blaming' and may be used to explain differences between people as being 'their own fault' when other factors need to be considered. For example, there is evidence that people from social class 4 and 5 suffer from poorer health than people who are in social class 1 and 2 and it is sometimes suggested that it is because they eat more fatty foods, smoke, drink alcohol and take little exercise. There is also evidence that people from social class 4 and 5 are more likely to have low birth-weight babies who are less likely to survive and that the mothers do not use the full range of ante natal services.

Activity 18

 Discuss with a friend how and why people in social class 4 and 5 may experience poorer health than those in social class 1 and 2. Discuss why the evidence that they have different lifestyles may be misleading and may lead to 'victim-blaming'.

COMMENT

 The evidence may be misleading because:

1 It creates the impression that people always have the resources to choose foods which are said to be 'healthy' i.e. low in fat, sugar, salt and high in the necessary nutrients (see Chapter 1, pages 7–10).

2 It does not really explain why this choice in diet may be made; for example, it may be that fatty foods or less 'nutritious' foods are cheaper and more readily available and indeed more filling, than high fibre, low fat and low sugar foods.

3 Public transport may be poor; people may have little or no access to a car which would take them to the larger out-of-town supermarkets.

4 Supermarkets are also very large in terms of floor space, which in itself may create problems for people with mobility difficulties.

5 They might not have access to information about 'healthy' diets.

6 It may also be due to other important issues such as housing, employment, childcare and finance taking priority over 'healthy' eating.

7 It may be that there are social reasons for the poorer health including high levels of stress, poor housing, low income and unemployment.

In looking only at dietary differences between people from different social classes, other important evidence may be missed. Similarly if you look at the evidence on low birth-weight babies and their mother's low attendance at ante-natal clinics and classes, it would be easy to conclude that increasing attendance might increase the level of birth weight and thus reduce the death rate. However there have been reports which suggest that while good ante-natal care is obviously important, so too is an adequate diet before and during pregnancy which can only be achieved through having an adequate income. Good housing and safe employment practices, plus a healthy lifestyle of not smoking or drinking alcohol, taking adequate rest and exercise may all contribute to the health and well-being of babies and their mothers.

It is therefore important to carefully weigh up any evidence or explanations which attempt to simplify the association between social class and ill-health.

Activity 19

 Jot down some reasons why some people's social class position may change or reasons why it may not be accurate.

COMMENT

Economic factors (such as periods of high unemployment in the country) may lead to people in one occupational group, e.g. engineers, to take another type of employment simply to earn a living. They could become drivers, labourers, shop workers etc., and so change social class.

Health factors may also influence someone's employment. A person who has developed a chronic health problem such as multiple sclerosis (MS), may have to take on part-time employment or work in their own home because of the unpredictable nature of the condition. Other people may be able to undertake employment despite having a physical condition such as MS, because the buildings in which they work have been adapted and improved for disabled employees: obstacles such as steps, heavy doors and poor signposting, which could prevent easy access, have been removed. The employer may allow work to be carried out either in the workplace or at home.

Social factors may also influence the social class classification: e.g. married women may be classified according to their husband's occupation. This means that the social class of women may not be accurate. Retired people are classified according to their past employment, or may be unclassified. The classification may give a clue as to certain aspects of their lifestyle but nothing can be taken for granted.

Other factors which may influence our lifestyle include our culture, race, and ethnic origin which will now be briefly discussed.

CULTURE

Our systems of beliefs, practices, customs, possessions, rituals, dress, language, spiritual beliefs and medical practices influence our lives. Different groups of people have different cultures although some aspects of culture may be shared. For example, some cultures share a disapproval of the use of alcohol or the eating of certain foods. Differences between groups of people need to be appreciated and respected. They play an important part in socialising people and determining their behaviour.

RACE

This factor refers to a number of differences in biological or physical attributes shared by a group of people. Often assumptions are made about people on the basis of biological or physical differences which, like the assumptions on class and gender, ignore the way in which society affects people in different ways.

ETHNIC ORIGIN

This is a term used to describe some common features or attributes of a subgroup in society. These shared features may include a language, a religion, a shared history, physical and cultural characteristics as well as a shared identity.

Assumptions are often made on the basis of people's culture, race and ethnicity. It has been found for example, that some people from different ethnic groups receive less help from social and health services when they are caring for dependent or elderly people. People may think that the dependent person's needs are being met by their 'family', meaning husband/wife/brothers/sisters/aunts/uncles/cousins. Some ethnic cultures firmly believe in the 'extended family' which supports and shares, but assumptions must not be made about the level of care needed from social services on this basis alone.

Families from any culture or ethnic group need to work to support themselves and so might not be available to care for a family member for reasons of time or location. Housing is often too small to accommodate the extended family adequately, and people may prefer to live separately in smaller households.

Amy's family would find it difficult to cope with caring for dependent relatives as they live in a three-bedroomed property and both parents also work. They may 'care about' their relatives and provide other kinds of support which would not be available from health and social services, but may not be in a position to 'care for' their relatives in terms of daily physical care. Joe's mother would not be in a position to provide care for dependent relatives in her present circumstances. She also lives far away from her parents, and would find it expensive and difficult either to travel or to telephone them. This does not mean that she does not 'care about' them (assuming of course that their relationship is good).

GENDER

This is a simple way of classifying people by describing them as either girls or boys, male or female, women or men. Although this may at first glance seem fairly self-explana-

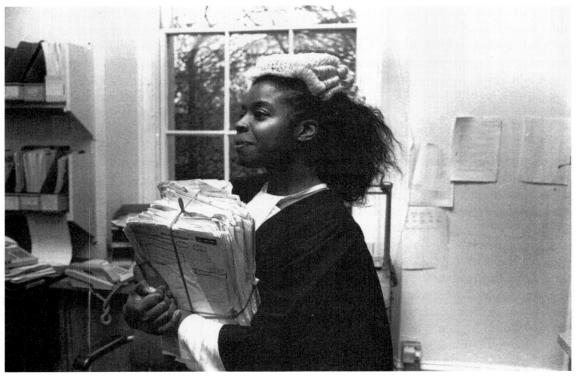

Figure 2.9   *Gradually, gender and racial barriers are being broken down in the professional world*

tory and based on biological differences, gender roles (the part which women and men, boys and girls play) in our society are affected by certain expectations. The way in which people greet the birth of a girl or a boy may be different: in some cultures, boys may be highly valued as a way of passing the family name.

Activity 20

Write down as many different examples as you can of treating girls and boys as you can think of.

COMMENT

- Boys and girls may be dressed differently from birth.
- They may be given different types of toys.
- Boys may be told 'big boys don't cry'.

- Girls and boys may be handled differently by their parents: e.g. boys are handled more roughly in play, and may be allowed to take more risks in play.
- They may be encouraged to undertake different household tasks as they get older.

Different families will bring up their children in different ways. These ideas represent a few examples of ways in which children may be treated differently depending upon their gender, but again it is important not to generalise.

Children are not just exposed to the attitudes of their parents; they are exposed to a range of people and situations which may influence how they feel about their own gender. They meet relatives, friends, teachers, members of the public, child minders, and they are exposed to the media. All of these contacts provide feedback to the child as to what is and what is not 'acceptable' behaviour, generally and specifically related to their gender. The child will also have its own ideas which will influence the way it reacts to being male or female.

You might find it useful to look at the television and films, and in newspapers and journals to see if there are different ways in which girls and boys, women and men are presented. The way in which we are brought up to behave as females and males is referred to as *role socialisation*. It is the process by which we are introduced to the norms, rules and social conventions or customs of the society in which we live. These gradually change and older relatives might tell you of ways in which they, as either female or male, were expected to behave and the sorts of work it was thought would be suitable for them, in their younger days.

Activity 21

Select at least six people of different ages, preferably one female and one male who are aged about 60 years old, one female and one male of about 40 years old, and one female and one male of about 20 years old.

Ask each of them what were acceptable toys, clothing and footwear, sporting activities, leisure pursuits, household tasks, employment, courting activities for boys and girls and men and women when they were growing up.

Compare the responses and identify those things that have changed and those that have remained the same.

COMMENT

You may have found that in some areas there is less distinction nowadays between accepted male and female behaviour, but that in other areas there has been little change.

Expectations and assumptions are often made about people simply on the grounds of their gender. Women may still be seen as naturally good at mothering and caring because they biologically and 'naturally' know how to do it. Women continue to be employed mainly in the caring sector as secretaries, nurses, cleaners and a range of other jobs, which are an extension of what some do in the home.

During World War II however, women did the majority of work in munitions factories building planes, working on the land, ploughing, planting, milking, haymaking, etc. Men have undertaken roles essentially seen as feminine, as they have entered for example the nursing profession. Some undertake full-time child care while their partners work in paid employment. However, it is not easy for either sex to adopt ways of behaving which are different from the norms. Men are expected to fight for their countries and provide for their families, while women are expected to care.

You may have found that in terms of career aspirations, women and men are now more able to choose a wider variety of possibilities than in the past. Amy's parents work in jobs which are now open to both men and women. Amy's sister wants to go to university and study to be a pharmacist. This might have not been an option for some of the people you interviewed who are in their 40s to 60s. There may be a social class or gender difference between people's career aspirations. Joanna may in the future take up a new form of employment, and undertake more training.

DISABILITY

Activity 22

Have a look around the built environment where you live and work. Make a note of the ways in which people with various disabilities are catered for in terms of mobility and access, communication aids for people with hearing loss, colour contrasts and audible signals for people with visual impairment.

COMMENT

In the past, able-bodied people have tended to design and construct our housing, access, roads, transport, shops, leisure services, theatres, cinemas, footpaths and other recreational facilities. Now people with disabilities are becoming involved in this type of design, with the result that these features are becoming more accessible to everyone.

Good examples of accessible environments can be found in leisure centres where planners have built in 'beach' entries to the swimming pools so that people wheel themselves into the water in special wheelchairs, and then are able to swim away. Dropped kerbs at crossing points, electronically operated doors are also examples of 'good' practice.

The more accessible the built environment, the greater the opportunities for people with disabilities and the 'temporary' able-bodied (at some time all of us may experience disability) to make the most use of that environment and to socialise with each other.

Of course our own attitudes to people who have a disability are important too. Positive attitudes encourage you to learn more about different forms of disability and how it affects individuals. They may also influence you to improve your understanding and skills in communication.

AGE

We said earlier that each of the families has members of different ages.

Activity 23

Have a look at Joe and Amy's family and write down their ages or approximate ages, and what you think society expects people to do at those ages.

Now write down some of the rules and laws which ensure that people at certain ages can or cannot do certain things.

COMMENT

Age is used as a rough guide as to whether or not we are capable of fulfilling a specific role in society. We are thought to be incapable of determining our sexuality under the age of 18 years old, and too young to enter any sexual relationship under 16 years, so there is a legal 'age of consent'. We are thought to be capable of working at 16 years of age, of voting at 18 years of age, and incapable of working at 65 years of age. You probably have found many other examples where age is the main reason on which a policy is based.

However in other countries and cultures, girls and boys of 12 years of age are able to form stable marital relationships, and people over the age of 65 years continue to work. This may lead you to think that perhaps age should only be used as a rough guide and that people's abilities are a better way of deciding what they can and cannot do.

Seven examples of differences between us which may influence our life experiences

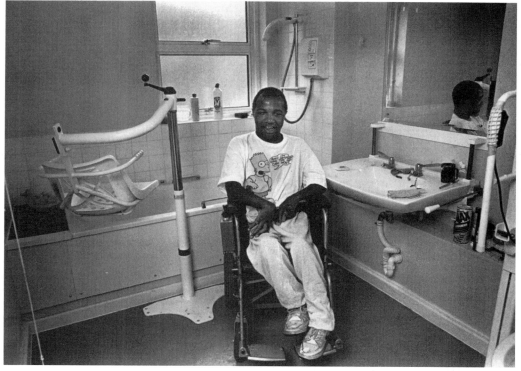

Figure 2.10   *An adapted bathroom enables this man to maintain his dignity and independence*

have been discussed so far: *social class, culture, race, ethnicity, gender, disability* and *age.* These examples show how positive and negative assumptions can be made about people based on limited information. Natural, biological and individual factors are often the easiest to understand and are the ones which are most commonly used to explain differences between people in society. However as you can see, they are not always as useful as they appear, as there are many different factors which influence the ways in which we lead our lives.

SOCIAL
CONVENTIONS

The explanations for individual differences are often based on common knowledge or common sense ideas and gradually become taken for granted. These categories are simple ways of grouping people together and finding common features which can be used to explain differences between them and the rest of the population. Having 'found' the differences, separate provisions, rules and laws may be developed to deal with them. Returning to the parts or roles we play in society, this section will look at roles, rules and social conventions within groups, to help you understand the ways in which we affect, and our behaviour is affected by, others in groups.

Taking part in society means that at different stages of our lives we may choose or be allocated roles such as a child, a member of a family, a student, a parent or an employee. In these different roles people are expected to behave in certain ways. Social scientists use the term 'role' to describe the expected pattern of behaviour of someone who holds a certain position in a group, an organisation or in society. The role holder has the status, e.g. a mother, which brings with it certain responsibilities and rights.

EXAMPLE

Refer back to the people in the two case studies on page 69 in this chapter. There was Amy (7 years old), her brother (aged 15 years), her older sister (17 years old), their mother, father and grandparents in case study 1. There was also Joe (aged 8) and his younger sister Jenni (aged 3) and their mother Joanna.

Each of these individuals in our society, is expected to behave in certain ways. They each have certain responsibilities and rights, which will vary depending upon the groups in which they find themselves and the society in which they live.

At three years of age, Jenni could go to a play school where she is a child in a group of other unrelated children. She has the right to the protection of those in whose charge she has been left, but she also has the responsibility of behaving well, within her abilities, to other children: i.e., play with them without undue aggression, share toys and share the attentions of the playgroup leaders. When she is at home, she is Joanna's daughter and can expect to have her physical, social and psychological needs met as far as possible, while her responsibilities will vary according to her mother's expectations of her at her age and abilities.

Joanna is a wife, even though she does not live with her husband. She can expect some financial support from him and he might expect to take part in their upbringing. He will expect Joanna to look after the children, making sure they are adequately cared for; she will probably expect him to work and provide support for them.

Each individual has roles and responsibilities within four main areas:

1 the family: husband, partner, wife, parent, child, grandparent.
2 the workplace as an employer or an employee, or in an educational setting as a member of a group, a student, a teacher.
3 recreational activities such as a Brownie or a Cub Scout: they may be participants, a leader or an organiser.
4 the community where they have other roles such as neighbours, friends, taxpayers, and voters.

Each of these roles may be separate and distinct, or they may overlap as individuals usually hold more than one role. Amy's father is a father to three children, a husband to his wife and a son to his parents (Amy's grandparents) as well as a brother to his siblings. He is an employee and a member of a religious group or sect.

Activity 24

Write down the different roles which you occupy in the family, in employment or in an educational setting, in recreational activities and in the community. Write down also the rights and responsibilities which are part of these roles.

COMMENT

You will have found that you have several roles. The rights and responsibilities attached to one role may be in harmony with those of another. However, sometimes when holding one role, you may experience some conflict; see Fig. 2.11.

EXAMPLE

Amy's mother works part-time as a nurse in a busy general practice. She has responsibilities at work for the health and well-being of

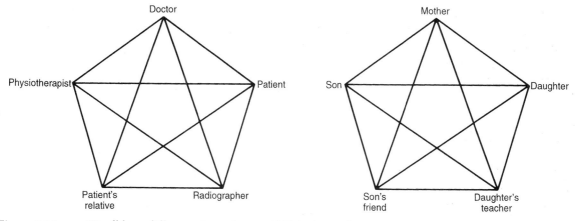

Figure 2.11   *We all have different roles and responsibilities in our lives*

patients who need her care. She has to keep up-to-date, reading journals, attending training, discussing care with others etc.

Amy may be unwell one day and need to stay at home. She is too young to be left, her father cannot have a day off, so Amy's mother will need to stay at home and care for Amy, unless a grandparent or other trusted person can be found. This means that some patients may be let down, and Amy's mother is worried about this.

Amy's mother might also need to read an important article about a new treatment she is expected to give. She wants to set aside some time to read, but her older son and daughter who are doing homework, want her attention. Her husband wants to talk about his day when he gets home from work.

Amy's mother will have to set boundaries to ensure that her needs are met too.

Changing roles and expectations

Did you find any conflicts in the different roles which you identified for yourself?

Amy too, will have expectations that her parents will take care of her, and these may be based on the ways in which men and women in Amy's social world organise their roles. These roles change over time, and are not static. In the past there were clearer divisions between the ways men and women behaved. On the whole, men had little to do with their children except to provide for them financially and discipline them; the expectations being that men worked long hours in employment. Women's work was mostly in the home, rearing children and doing housework.

Men and women's work both in the house and in the workplace have changed and are continuing to change. This means that Amy's father may take a day off to look after Amy when she is unwell, just as her mother may. Her father's job may be undertaken at home using the latest computer technology, therefore the conflict of roles (employer, mother/father to Amy) may not be so acute.

Amy's mother's employers will also expect her to be at work and undertake her role in a way which is expected of a nurse. There are rules and social conventions within which roles are acted out. Nurses share certain ideas, theories and expectations, which affect the way in which they behave, and expect each other to behave. If nurses act outside of these rules and norms, they may be seen as unusual or deviant, and may be punished in some way. Some of the rules and norms are enshrined by the profession in a Code of Conduct. Any breaches in this Code of Conduct could mean that the nurse is unable to practice as a nurse.

Some of the rules and social conventions are not very obvious, but nevertheless are accepted and understood within certain social groups. When you are living in a family, it may be an unspoken rule that talking about family affairs outside the family is not done. If a family member does say something which they should not, to someone outside the family, the family might let the member 'save face' and accept that it was a slip of the tongue, or they may 'tell off' the member, thus reinforcing the rules.

These social rules and conventions are positive in that they act as guides and standards for acceptable behaviour and let society members know what is unacceptable. They help us make sense of society and to anticipate and cope with interactions within the different groups and organisations to which we belong. There may also be negative effects, as in some social groups it may be the norm to smoke, to steal or to be aggressive. Group members may be required to conform to the rules and norms regardless of whether they are positive or negative, and may indeed not be seen as such within the group.

You may have seen films about 'undercover' police who disguise themselves and join a criminal group in order to discover their actions, identify the ringleaders and find sufficient evidence to convict them. In order to maintain their disguise, they have to behave like criminals. If they behaved like the police, they would soon be found out and would therefore be unsuccessful in their mission.

There are other groups in society who have different standards from the majority population but are clearly not criminal, simply pursuing a different lifestyle. These groups include gypsies and New Age Travellers, who prefer to live in caravans, rather than houses. They may remain on one campsite or be nomadic, and they may pursue different types of occupations such as recycling materials or working in agriculture. Laws such as the Criminal Justice and Public Order Act 1994 prevent them from moving about freely and try to control their lifestyle. Certain groups may challenge these laws in order to help people continue their preferred lifestyle. The challenges to this and other laws by social groups through protests and demonstrations prove that there are a variety of opinions to be taken into account, and the demonstration of these opinions may bring about changes in society.

The lifestyle of some groups may be little understood by others and may lead to misunderstandings. However within these minority groups, people have roles and responsibilities, norms and social conventions which help to govern the behaviour of their members. While groups in society have norms which are not fully understood or acceptable to other groups, it must be agreed that we live in a multi-cultural society and that we need to live together, in harmony, with these differences.

Activity 25

Having looked at social class, and discussed how occupation and other social divisions may affect health, and having looked at roles, norms and social conventions, it is important to consider ways in which these may affect health.

Pause now, look back over the chapter so far, and make notes about the ways in which these characteristics may affect health.

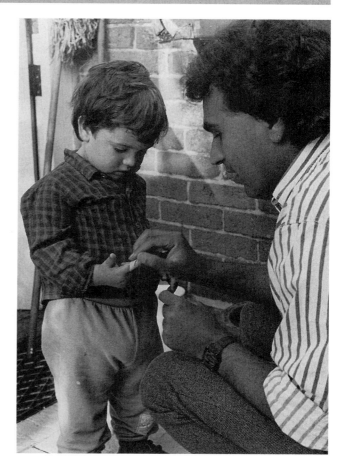

Figure 2.12   *Childcare is no longer seen as being the sole responsibility of the mother*

COMMENT

ⓘ There are a number of important points which need to be remembered from this section:

1 The term 'family' does not necessarily mean, mother, father and two children living in the same household. In a society made up of many groups, there are several different ways of organising living arrangements, some of which may include mother, father and children, but many which do not.

2 Roles, norms and social conventions differ in family groups depending upon culture and the society in which the groups live. These roles, norms and social conventions may change over time.

3 Employment, income and social policies affect the health of people in different social classes in various ways. People in lower social classes often have poorer health. This is not necessarily due to their lifestyle but to low wages, low welfare benefits, poorer housing and less access to health services. Looking solely at 'lifestyle' may lead to victim-blaming rather than looking at wider social issues.

4 Culture, race, ethnic origin, gender, age

and disability influence individual choices which might affect health, but so do the wider social issues such as discrimination, which may prevent people from participating fully and equally in society.

5 The roles we play in society are governed by norms and social conventions, although we undertake those roles in our own personal style, changing the roles as society changes. Physical, mental and social well-being are affected by the pressures which are exerted on individuals in society, to conform.

Summary

This section has taken a fairly wide view about the ways in which our well-being may be affected by social factors:

- health depends on our lifestyle but it is also affected by factors outside our control, such as the social class to which we belong, and the way in which our culture, race and ethnicity is perceived by others.

- social expectations and pressures influence the way in which we act out our roles. Women and men tend to be concentrated in certain occupations, but society is constantly changing: men and women are able to challenge these expectations and pressures.

- society's perception and response to our needs. Where there is adequate awareness, the environment may be hospitable and accessible, enabling us to move around and participate fully in society. On the other hand, it may be difficult to take on particular roles in society, if that society is not willing to improve access for disabled people. It may be difficult for a person with disabilities to be a student, if they are faced with poor transport, poor access and inadequate facilities and resources.

- identify ways in which you are responsible for promoting your health and well-being and that of others.

- other organisations such as government also have a responsibility for funding and providing services which will directly affect our health.

3

HEALTH AND SOCIAL CARE SERVICES

AIMS AND OBJECTIVES

The aims of this chapter are to enable you to:

- know why health and social services exist and describe the different needs they try to meet.

- explain the organisation of statutory health and social care services.

- describe the health and social care services provided by non-statutory and independent sectors and explain the ways they are funded.

- describe the forms of health and social care provided by informal carers.

- outline the main laws which govern the way the services are provided and delivered.

- explain how a person in need can have access to help.

- understand the meaning of client rights and appreciate the importance of confidentiality.

- describe the main jobs that exist within health and social care services, and what these jobs involve.

The provision of health and social services

WHY DO WE HAVE HEALTH AND SOCIAL CARE SERVICES?

Can you imagine a baby or young child left to live entirely alone? They would not last very long without any support from other people. Adults sometimes joke about living on a desert island, but in practice we soon realise how much we all depend on one another.

We all have needs. Some last throughout our lives, e.g. the need for food, clothes, warmth, shelter (i.e. housing), security and companionship. Some needs are less general. Certain people have mental or physical disabilities, loss of sight or hearing, learning difficulties or mobility problems. These may be a result of illness or accident or may have been present from birth. Other needs occur at particular stages of life, for example during pregnancy, early childhood, bereavement or old age.

Activity 1

Think about an area you know well, perhaps the estate in which you live, or the streets through which you walk to get to college. Imagine yourself knocking on the door of each house or flat, and finding out about the people living at each address.

Make a list of these imaginary families and their needs.

Here are some examples to help you:

- a family whose father is unemployed
- an old man with very poor eyesight, living alone
- a mother who is in hospital having just had her first baby
- a family with a teenage son who is suspected to be taking drugs
- a woman who has just discovered that she has a lump in her breast
- a 16-year-old boy about to leave his school for handicapped pupils
- a family where the mother has just been discharged from hospital after a major operation

COMMENT

Of course, you will probably come across many families without any very obvious 'problems' or needs! For the sake of this exercise, we are examining many experiences that only happen from time to time in most families. It might be a good idea also to compare notes with others in your group.

As you have thought about many different circumstances and needs, you might begin to think about the sorts of care that might be appropriate to meet the needs, and who might be able to give this care.

WHAT ARE HEALTH AND SOCIAL CARE SERVICES?

As children, most of our basic needs are met within the family, by our parents. One or both of them go out to work to earn money to buy the things needed for themselves and their family.

The parents' role is to care for their children, making sure they have the necessary food, clothes, warmth, rest and exercise. Parents are the first teachers children have. The mother or father looks after the children during minor illnesses, and tries to keep them healthy by giving them a proper diet and by protecting them from accident. At the same time, the family provides companionship, social stimulation and emotional support. The home is the place where family members find someone to share their interests, to talk to when they are upset or have problems at school or at work.

Parents may be helped in all this by grandparents, aunts, uncles, or other members of the 'extended family' if they live nearby. No family can, however, be completely self sufficient. In Britain today, there are often few members of the extended family who are free and live near enough to give regular help.

Even in cultures where it is the tradition for the family to take as much responsibility as possible for the needs of its members, there is a place for care and support from outside the family. This may come from 'informal' helpers, friends, neighbours, local shopkeepers, employers etc., who may offer advice, information and practical support.

Mostly, though, extra help will be sought from 'professionals': i.e. people who are

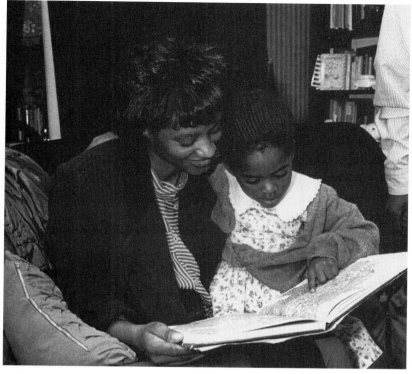

Figure 3.1   *Parents have the primary responsibility of caring for their child's health and well-being*

trained, qualified, and paid to give support of various kinds. In all, even underdeveloped, societies, there are some such people; e.g. the doctor, the midwife, the school teacher, the priest.

In the past, these positions were filled by private individuals who had particular skills and who established themselves or were appointed by the local community, to fulfil certain functions. In most modern westernised societies, however, the state has taken responsibility for providing what it considers to be the necessary services.

The state has always been responsible for such things as law and order, defence, and more recently for regulation of employment and management of the economy, but the twentieth century in Britain saw the development of the 'welfare state'. The state became responsible for the direct and immediate wel-fare of its citizens. It did this by setting up institutions which we call 'social services' and 'health services'.

The focus of social service and of health service provision is on family groups and on the individuals within these groups. Social policy generally aims to give everyone equal opportunities and so enhance welfare or well-being.

Statutory services

Social services provided by the state are described as 'statutory' or official services, and a state with many statutory services can be called a 'welfare state'. Services are provided by the state through central government departments, through departments of local authorities, or via special boards. The way statutory services are organised is described later on in this chapter.

Non-statutory services

Organised services not provided directly by the state are called 'non-statutory' or independent. Some are 'voluntary' organisations (i.e. non-profit making, often charitable bodies). A voluntary organisation is an association or society that has come into existence of its own accord; it has been created by its members rather than being created by the state. This does not mean that all its members work voluntarily. There will probably be many unpaid volunteers, but especially in larger organisations, the staff will mainly be paid employees. Examples of voluntary organisations are Age Concern, the British Red Cross, and the Women's Royal Voluntary Service.

Other non-statutory organisations may be private, i.e. run as a business, to make a profit. Nursing and residential homes, agencies delivering home care, and nursery schools are examples of private provision of social or health care. There are also many self-employed individuals, e.g. offering child minding, cleaning, foster care.

It is important to remember that much social care (and to a lesser extent health care) continues to be provided by 'informal' unpaid carers. These include parents, children, friends and neighbours and local support groups. They may help with physical care for disabled people, child minding, shopping, transport, gardening, provision of meals and many other needs.

There are different views and political opinions as to what should be the proper balance between services provided by the state and those left to the individual or to voluntary bodies. Equality, individual responsibility and choice are only some of many relevant considerations.

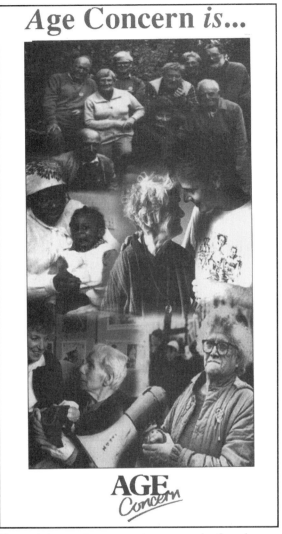

Figure 3.2   *Age concern is an example of a voluntary organisation with active local branches*

Activity 2

Go back to your imaginary street and the needs you discovered there. How are these varied needs met? What help is available and through which organisations and individuals?

Appropriate help may be of many different kinds. Go through the list and write down the sort of help the people concerned might welcome. Is the help they need to do with:

- finance
- practical chores (cleaning, shopping, laundry, decorating, gardening etc.)
- health
- housing (including facilities or equipment)
- education
- employment
- loneliness
- safety
- advice or counselling
- other factors?

Activity 3

 So who gives help?
Do this exercise with a partner or in a small group:

Make two columns, and write down (in any order) as many people as you can think of, who might be involved in meeting the needs you have just listed.

Use the first column for people who are unpaid (e.g. friends and family or others who give voluntary help through an organisation).

Use the second column for paid, 'professional' workers (e.g. home help, nurse). Some of these helpers visit people in their own homes. Others work in an office or centre and their 'clients' (i.e. those who use their help) visit them at their place of work.

As you read through the next section, see how many of the services mentioned, you have already thought about.

THE STRUCTURE OF HEALTH AND CARE SERVICES

Levels of care

Care is provided at different points of delivery:

PRIMARY CARE

This term is used to describe care, often preventative, delivered in the community. It is usually the initial point of contact, for example with a GP, social worker, health visitor.

SECONDARY CARE

This is when care, often curative, is provided in a specialist setting like a hospital or a day centre; e.g. a chiropody clinic in a hospital, or a mental health group. It is important to realise that one service may provide, at different times, both primary and secondary care. A paramedic giving treatment at the scene of an accident is an example of primary care, whereas an ambulance driver in the ambulance service collecting a client for physiotherapy treatment at a hospital is an example of secondary care.

TERTIARY CARE

This is the term given to care provided through long-term rehabilitation, e.g. inpatient hospital treatment or residential care of people with severe learning disabilities.

Health services

In Britain, most aspects of health care come within the scope of the National Health Service (NHS), which was set up in 1948, after the National Health Service Act was passed in 1946. One of its aims was to make health care equally available to everyone.

It is organised under the central government Department of Health (see Fig. 3.2). In England, the NHS is divided into 14 regional health authorities. Wales constitutes a single region. Each region contains a number of district health authorities. At district level there are community health councils (CHCs) in order to represent the views of the general public (the consumers). In

Scotland there are 15 health boards, and in Northern Ireland 4 health boards.

Hospitals are a major part of the NHS and most people at some point in their lives experience hospital care either as an out-patient or as an in-patient. Attendance is either by referral from a GP or through an Accident and Emergency department. Treatment is free at the point at which it is received, its cost having been subsidised by payment of National Insurance contributions which everyone in employment is required to make.

There are also some private hospitals,

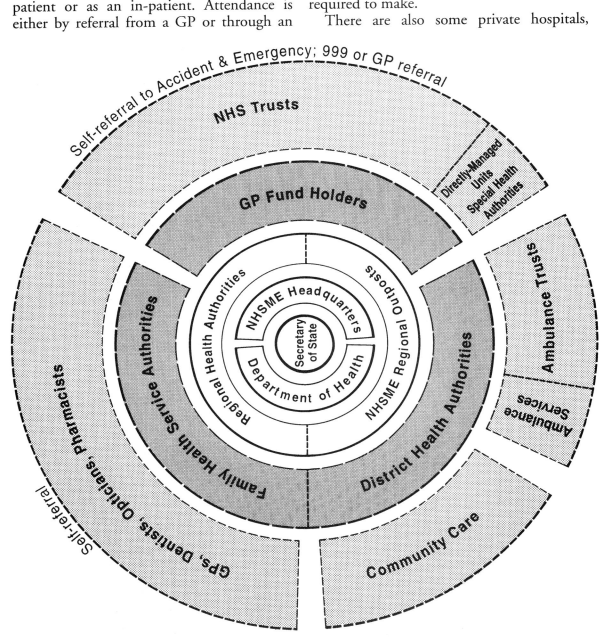

Figure 3.3   *The structure of the NHS*

which are outside the National Health Service. Patients using these hospitals have to pay for their own treatment, although many belong to private insurance schemes which cover the cost.

Other important work of the NHS comes under the heading of 'community health services'. This includes health education, antenatal and child health clinics, family planning and school health services.

There are over 30,000 General Practitioners (GPs) in Britain, and these are usually the first point of contact for patients. GPs are independent and self employed, but are contracted to their family health services authority (FHSA).

Other health professionals who form part of the 'primary care team' include district nurses, health visitors, community psychiatric nurses, midwives, chiropodists, speech therapists. Dentists can choose whether to work privately or to have an arrangement with the FHSA, whereby they see patients under the NHS.

In 1990 the NHS and Community Care Act was passed. Among its key objectives were:

- to make services more responsive to the consumer
- to give patients the widest possible choice of service
- to raise standards of care.

THE SOCIAL SECURITY SYSTEM

The Department of Social Security (DSS) administers most of the financial help avail-

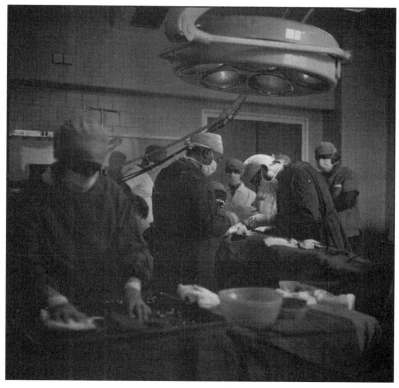

Figure 3.4   *We may all need hospital care at some stage in our lives*

able to people with disabilities. The former Department of Health and Social Security was split into two separate departments (the Department of Health and the Department of Social Security) in 1988.

The DSS provides cash benefits to people with no income or a low income, those with special needs and to people who have contributed to the National Insurance Scheme. Local authorities administer housing and council tax benefits and education benefits. The NHS administers health benefits, e.g. free prescriptions, although the benefits agency is responsible for the means test. Employers are responsible for the payment of some benefits, e.g. Statutory Sickness Pay.

One group of benefits is based on National Insurance Contributions ('stamps'), e.g. sickness benefit and retirement pension. Income support and housing benefit, on the other hand, are *means-tested*. Entitlement depends on a person's income, savings, age, size of family, and other personal circumstances. *Non-means-tested* benefits are paid regardless of income or savings, provided the person qualifies by showing that they have the relevant need. Examples are child benefit, attendance allowance for people over 65 who need help with personal care, and disability living allowance for people under 65 needing help with personal care or with getting around.

SOCIAL SERVICES

A social service can be defined as a service provided by the community to help those in need. Services can include:

- financial benefits
- health care
- education
- employment services
- housing

- planning
- youth services
- probation
- after care
- local welfare services (sometimes called personal social services).

Social services departments are local authority departments (county council or metropolitan borough), whose responsibility is mainly for personal social services. These departments employ social workers and other categories of workers to carry out their duties.

Social workers

The role of social workers is

- to help their clients to understand better the nature of their problems
- to give support
- to advise clients on how best to deal with their problems.

The extent to which social workers specialise in particular sorts of problems (e.g. mental health, child abuse) has varied over the years, but in general, all social workers seek to deal with an individual's problems in the context of the family.

The general public does not always understand very well the role of social workers. They often deal with very sensitive issues, such as child abuse. They can be accused on the one hand of not intervening soon enough to prevent a child suffering abuse, and on the other hand of over-interference with parental rights. Social workers are sometimes disparagingly referred to as 'do-gooders' by some people who nostalgically look back to a time when it was believed that families and local communities provided all the support needed without recourse to 'professionals'. Social workers have to undertake several years of full-time training in order to qualify.

OTHER OCCUPATIONS

Local authorities also employ people in other positions such as home carers, cooks, child minders, drivers, day care assistants etc., who are trained, but not to such a high level. There are also ancillary professions such as occupational therapists who work in social service departments. (Equally, some social workers are employed within the health service.)

Legislation

The NHS and Community Care Act 1990 referred to above greatly extended the responsibilities of social service departments. The main aim of 'Community Care' is to help people live in their own community, as independently as possible in their own homes. The law says that each social service department must find out what sort of help is needed by people living in their area, who are finding it difficult to cope because of age, disability, or mental health problems. The social workers then arrange to make 'contracts' for the necessary services to be provided by private companies, voluntary (non-profit making) organisations, or by the social services department itself.

Services are offered to people with physical disabilities, mental health problems or learning disabilities, older people, families with children, and young people. Some people are referred to the social worker by other professionals such as doctors or nurses. Others contact them directly, or a friend or informal carer makes the contact on behalf of the client. There are offices or advice centres belonging to the social services department in each local area. Once a referral has been made, a community care worker will

meet the client to make an assessment of what the needs are, and to decide what services would best meet the needs, taking into account the wishes of the client and his or her carers, as well as the opinions of other professionals. Of course, there are very many people asking for help, and a limit to the finance and the services available, so these will necessarily go to those in greatest need.

Services which may be arranged include the following:

- day care at a centre with organised activities
- personal care: help with bathing, dressing, etc.
- respite care: a short stay in a residential home
- meals on wheels
- help with household tasks
- work training
- special equipment
- occupational therapy
- counselling and support
- information and advice
- long-term residential care
- subsidised holidays
- transport

You will see that while the health service and social services are separate structures, there may be much overlap involved in the needs of a particular client. Professionals from the two departments therefore need to work closely together if the individual client is to receive services geared to his or her particular needs, regardless of the employing authority of those providing the care.

Since the implementation of Community Care legislation, there has been much controversy about the funding of services. This has arisen from the financial shortfall some local authorities have suffered in making provision for the needs they have identified in their area. In addition, the move away from providing long-term care for elderly people

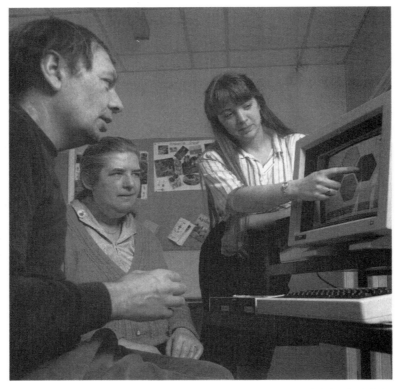

Figure 3.5 *Occupational therapists help people to learn or re-learn skills needed for daily life*

within the NHS (which is non-means-tested) towards provision in nursing or residential homes (for which financial assistance *is* means-tested) has been much disputed, not least by those who have had to sell property in order to fund their care.

NON-STATUTORY SERVICES

Many of the types of service mentioned above, as part of health and social services, are also provided by private and voluntary organisations. For example:

1 Day centres are run by bodies like Age Concern, Scope (Mencap), National Children's Society, the Alzheimer's Disease Society, etc.
2 Play groups and family centres are held on many church premises
3 Private counselling agencies.

Residential care homes and nursing homes are increasingly being provided both by voluntary (non-profit making) bodies and private (business) companies.

INFORMAL CARERS

Much care and support is given to individuals and to families by informal, unpaid carers. If this were not the case, the already over-stretched statutory services would be under an unbearable strain.

There are many people caring at home for members of their family with often severe physical and mental disabilities, and this care may be provided over many years. Carers of elderly people are often themselves elderly and not in good health. At the other end of the scale, quite young children are often helping substantially to care for disabled parents or brothers or sisters.

For these informal carers, the availability of support services, such as respite care, day care, transport, sitters, etc., is vital. Many local areas also have informal support groups providing much needed assistance with, for example, transport, shopping, gardening. Much time is given by volunteers within these schemes.

All carers now have the right to a separate local authority assessment of their own needs, under the Carer's (Recognition and Services) Act 1995.

Activity 4

Go for a walk-about! Take a notebook and walk around your nearest town centre, making a note of any buildings, offices, centres, that seem to have to do with the social, practical, health needs you have been thinking about. If you are not sure, write the name down anyway, and find out from your tutor afterwards what goes on in the place concerned. Have a look, too, at notice boards in shops, libraries or post offices. These may also give you some clues as to what services are available in the area.

COMMENT

Compare notes with others in your group. Together you will probably discover some services you didn't know about before; there may be many others that you still don't know about.

So, how can you find out some more? We shall come back to the availability of infor-mation later on, but for the moment, try using the telephone directory, or Yellow Pages. Look up health services, social services, and Department of Social Security.

HOW ARE THE SERVICES PAID FOR?

Different types of services are funded in different ways. Where the state has set up statutory services, the government makes financial provision for them by allocating money either directly, or to regional or local authorities for them to administer. The necessary money has to be raised by government through taxation of its citizens.

Non-statutory service providers may receive grants from the state, if the government sees the organisation as providing a necessary and appropriate service to complement its own provision. Recent legislation has tended to shift the balance from central and local government making a lot of direct provision of services to meet health and social care needs, towards their 'purchasing' more services from either voluntary or private organisations or individuals. One example of this change has been allowing GPs to hold their own funds and to choose where to purchase the services (e.g. hospital treatment) needed by their patients. The 'providers' now include hospital trusts and community trusts.

Similarly, social service departments of local authorities now mostly purchase the residential and day care services for people they have assessed as needing these, rather than provide these establishments for themselves. 'Contracts' are set up which lay down the responsibility of the provider to give a suitable service and of the purchaser to pay at an agreed rate. The individuals concerned will be part of this contract, and according to the type of service, and their means, will be required to contribute towards the cost of care.

Voluntary organisations also do fund raising, and may receive donations towards their financial needs. Health and social care insurance has also come to play a much larger part in enabling individuals to buy the care they need.

Meeting the needs of different clients

WHO ARE THE SERVICES FOR?

The simple answer to this question is that they are for everyone! Most people need to use health services at one time or another. They visit their GP with minor ailments, use the ambulance service after an accident, and can be referred to a hospital as an out-patient or in-patient for medical or surgical treatment.

Social care services are also available for everyone, but in practice there are certain groups of people for whom services are particularly provided:

1 Because of special family circumstances, e.g. bereavement or abuse, children may need foster care, residential care, or day nursery provision.
2 Adolescents may have problems at home, and need counselling or practical help.
3 Mentally and physically disabled people may need considerable practical, financial and social work help to enable them to lead as full and normal lives as possible. Some will need long-term residential or nursing care.
4 While most old people stay in their own homes, they may need much support to make this possible; e.g. home care, practical aids, meals on wheels, day care, respite care to give their family carer a break. A minority will become so frail that they will need permanent residential or nursing home care.

HOW CAN THE SERVICES BE OBTAINED?

As we have already seen, there are different ways in which people can be referred to health and social care services. A professional, for example a GP, may refer someone to another professional, perhaps a physiotherapist, social worker, or hospital consultant. Sometimes a person makes a *self referral*, e.g., he decides to go and see a dentist, a Citizens Advice Bureau or a social worker.

Referral by others is when someone concerned about another person, makes contact on their behalf with a professional. For example, a neighbour may refer an elderly person who is wandering, to a social worker; or a head teacher may refer a pupil to an educational psychologist. Referral by emergency services could be as the result of an injury which is thought to be non-accidental.

Of course, for individuals to be referred, or to refer themselves, they must know what help is available, where it is to be found, and how they can get in touch with the appropriate people.

Scenario

At the beginning of term, you discover that a new student, Beverley, has joined your course at college. You find that she and her family have just moved into the area, and that she lives not far from you. One day, Beverley looks worried, and tells you that her three-year-old sister is ill. You ask if the child has seen a doctor, and Beverley tells you that her mother is not sure how to get in touch with a doctor.

Activity 5

Imagine that you decide to go home with Beverley and try and help. What information and help will you give the family about contacting a doctor? Jot down your ideas before reading the next section.

COMMENT

Names and addresses of doctors can be found at the Citizens Advice Bureau, or in libraries. Every person resident in this country has a right to receive free medical treatment under the National Health Service. He or she must ask at the doctor's surgery to be 'registered', i.e. added to his or her list of patients; normally doctors will accept on to their lists people living within a reasonable distance of the practice.

Activity 6

Go back to your 'walk about' exercise. Get hold of a map of your local area (or draw one for yourself). Using what you found out about the local services and what you have just been reading, mark on the map the offices and centres, hospitals and surgeries, and any other relevant buildings where services are to be found. Starting from where you yourself live, or choosing the home of someone you know, make a list of which services are:

- within half a mile
- within two miles
- within five miles
- further than five miles away

COMMENT

What conclusions do you draw from this? What is the public transport like in the area? Which service would it be very difficult or impossible for someone to get to without their own transport? Bearing in mind opening times of clinics, etc., and times of buses, would there be a lot of waiting around involved?

This brings us to the topic of access to information and to services which are there to help people.

Activity 7

1 Choose one of the client groups about which we have been thinking, e.g. an elderly frail person, a family with young children, or a physically disabled person.

2 Imagine you are the person concerned, and that you are trying to find out about what help may be available to you. Set out to gather as much information as possible. The library, Citizens Advice Bureau, Post Office, doctors' surgeries, may be good places to start.

3 Ask for any leaflets available, both at these general sources of information, and from the services themselves.

4 When you have gathered as much information as you can, discuss the following with your group:

   a Would the person you are imagining yourself to be, have been able to get to the place they needed to go to?
   b Is there a bus or train near it?
   c Does the building have easy access e.g. ramps for disabled people or help for mothers pushing prams?

d Look at the leaflets critically. Would most people be able to understand them easily and know what they had to do next?

e Is it made clear how a person can contact a social worker?

f What if the family is from another country, e.g. Bangladesh, and speaks little English? Are there leaflets available in different languages? Is the help of interpreters offered?

g Could you fill in a benefit application form without help?

h What about the elderly person who says that he doesn't want charity and refuses to apply for benefits to which he is entitled?

Client rights

Every person has a right to benefit from the services which are appropriate to his or her needs. What, in practice, does this mean?

- You must know the service exists.
- You must understand how to apply for the service.
- You must be able to contact the relevant person or get hold of the appropriate application form.
- You may need access to a telephone or transport.
- Information leaflets need to be in a language and use words you can understand.
- You have a right not to be discriminated against in receiving health or care services on account of race, sex, age, disability or for any other reason.

This may mean you need to have the support of someone like an interpreter, if the health or social service does not use your first language. A person with learning difficulties or with mental health problems, may need to have an 'advocate', i.e. someone (not a professional) who will speak up on his or her behalf, e.g. in a 'case conference' at which decisions are being made about his or her future, and who will act as an advocate if necessary.

Increasingly, health and social services produce written documents which list users' rights, i.e. what service they can expect to receive from the organisation or individual concerned. Examples are the Patients' Charter or a Residents' Charter which may form part of the contract for someone entering a residential care or nursing home.

There is legislation which service-givers must comply with: e.g. the Sex Discrimination Act 1975 and the Race Relations Act 1976. Over and above this, the responsibility not only to provide the service but to make this truly accessible to the client, must rest with the professionals concerned. See Chapter 4, for further discussion of discrimination in care settings.

Scenarios

1 An elderly Asian man is assessed as needing meals on wheels and day care. He refuses both because he is offered food which his religion forbids him to eat. Is this discrimination, and how should the social workers concerned deal with this situation?

2 A disabled person living at home needs help to get ready for bed each night. She is offered the services of a home care assistant but is told that because of other commitments, the carer has to come at 8 pm each evening. Is this acceptable help? Does it allow the client an appropriate degree of choice and dignity?

3 An elderly woman living at home alone keeps falling. She does not always remember to turn off the cooker after she has used it. Her neighbours are worried about her safety, but she insists that she does not want to move into a residential home.

What are her rights? What about her neighbours' rights?

COMMENT

ⓘ Can you think of any more examples of how a service may exist, but not meet the clients' rights to make decisions for themselves or to be treated with dignity?

CONFIDENTIALITY

A professional person providing social or health care, e.g. a social worker or a care assistant, gets to know a lot of very personal and private information about their clients, and may also be involved in giving quite intimate personal care. It is essential that this information is kept confidential and is not discussed without the client's permission.

Of course, some information may need to be passed on from one professional to another; e.g. a social worker may want to refer the client to another worker, such as a nurse, an occupational therapist or a residential care home manager. However, this passing on of information *must* be with the client's consent and knowledge.

Most social service departments now have clear procedures for clients to be able to see any records that are being kept on them, and it is important that clients are made aware of their rights in this matter.

A client needs to have confidence that any conversations between himself or herself and the social worker or care worker will be kept completely confidential. Close relationships may well develop between the client and the worker. These relationships can and should be friendly and informal but still remain professional.

Investigating jobs in health and social care

We have seen that there are very many different people working in many different organisations, whose job it is to provide health and social care. All of them are dealing with individuals and families, but they bring a variety of skills and experience, and have undergone education and training at different levels. Their work patterns and working conditions also vary.

Some of the main jobs in health and social care are described below, covering both those who provide care, and those who support professional carers.

THE IMPACT OF COMMUNITY CARE

You will notice a great many references to the move towards community care, and the impact that this has had on the provision of health and caring services. Community care has developed since the 1990 Act to encourage the provision of care in two distinct ways:

1 Care provided in people's own homes by a range of health and social services, such as district nurses and care assistants.

2 Care by health and social service workers in residential accommodation, which is small scale and placed within the local community. Examples are hostels for people with learning difficulties, and Old People's homes.

The great majority of jobs within the health and caring services have been affected by the development of community care. However, jobs relating particularly to this type of care include: district nurses, health visitors, GPs, occupational therapists, those running day centres, social workers and care assistants.

In the following pages you will find out more about the jobs listed below:

Health carers:

- General Practitioner
- Hospital consultant
- Osteopath
- Dentist
- Radiographer
- Physiotherapist
- Occupational therapist
- Optician

- Registered general nurse – adult nursing
- Registered general nurse – mental health nursing
- Health visitor
- District nurse
- Practice nurse
- Midwife

Social carers:

- Social worker
- Counsellor
- Care assistant

Support services:

- Clinic assistant or manager
- Administrative staff
- Clerical staff

Activity 8

Using the checklist above, select two jobs in each of the categories: health carers, social carers, support staff. List three points which you think stereotype each role, such as working hours, or day-to-day tasks, for each. Then compare your notes with the descriptions below.

HEALTH CARERS

General Practitioners

DAY-TO-DAY WORK

The great majority of doctors work in general practice, where they treat clients living within a geographical area. The term 'general' is used as these doctors deal with every illness or other condition brought to them by the client. Even if they cannot treat the

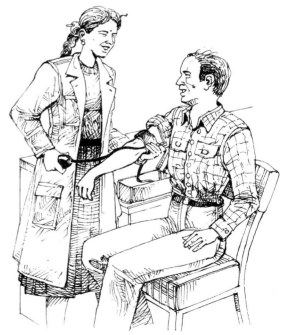

Figure 3.6   *A GP deals with all kinds of medical complaints*

condition themselves, they are still the first point of contact for the client. In these cases, the GP will refer the patient on to a consultant who is a specialist in the particular problem area.

The General Practitioner's role also includes prevention of disease and helping clients stay in good health. An increasing number of GPs work under contracts where their income is set according to the number and type of clients treated. These GPs must reach government targets, e.g. for inoculation and primary health checks (such as cervical smear testing), before receiving the full amount of money.

Most GPs hold surgeries morning and evening, and will visit clients who need to remain in their own homes during the day. Traditionally, GPs had the satisfaction of seeing patients in the context of their family, and of providing long-term care, sometimes getting to know different generations of the same family. Increasingly however, GPs work in group practices, so that someone, not necessarily the named doctor you are registered with, is always available. This also means that night visits are shared among a greater number of doctors, and may be carried out by 'locums' or relief doctors.

Hospital consultants

Doctors working in hospital, by contrast, tend to treat patients over shorter periods, though many people have chronic conditions which means they have to visit out-patient departments over a long period. Also unlike GPs, hospital consultants tend to specialise in one particular area of medicine. For instance, they may deal especially with sick children (paediatricians), problems of internal body systems (endocrinologists), or heart ailments (cardiologists). Most consultants also work long hours, and are on call at night and weekends.

Other types of doctor

Medicine is one of the most varied professions. As well as GPs and hospital specialists, many doctors work in industry as occupational health physicians, in the navy and armed forces, or in government service. Others carry out full-time research into new methods of medical practice. New discoveries are always making their impact on medical practice, e.g. newly developed drugs have enabled Parkinson's disease sufferers to live longer. As well as drugs, there is new research in areas such as electronics, nuclear physics, genetics and molecular biology.

CAREER ROUTES AND TRAINING FOR ALL DOCTORS

Learning to be a doctor is one of the longest and most expensive of any course of training. A science background is needed, and all medical schools ask for an A level or AS level in chemistry (or physical science). Most then require two other science A levels.

Traditional medical school courses are made up of two years of pre-clinical learning, covering subjects such as anatomy, physiology, biochemistry, psychology, medical sociology, basic pathology (knowledge of diseases) and pharmacology (knowledge of drugs). Another three years are then taken up with a clinical course, where the medical student works in hospital wards with a 'firm' or team of qualified doctors, usually including two consultants, a senior registrar, registrar, a senior house officer, and junior house officer.

Newer courses are now being developed where students mix the pre-clinical and clinical training to a much greater extent. More time is now also given to developing communication skills, carrying out practical clinical tasks, and studying a few subjects in greater depth.

A sixth year must then be spent as a junior

house officer in a general hospital before the medical student can apply for full registration with the General Medical Council. Any doctor who breaches the GMC code of practice during his or her career will be 'struck off the register', and so be unable to continue working as a doctor.

After these six years and further training, a registered doctor will then be fully qualified to work as a General Practitioner. In order however to specialise as a consultant, more study and exams are involved, together with further experience in the relevant hospital ward. Specialisms include:

- Anaesthetics
- Accident and Emergency medicine
- Cardiology
- Dermatology
- Endocrinology
- General (Internal) Medicine
- Geriatric Medicine
- Neurology
- Paediatrics
- Renal medicine
- Ophthalmology
- Obstetrics and Gynaecology
- Pathology
- Psychiatry
- Radiology
- Radiotherapy and Oncology
- Surgery

For further information, write to:
Careers Division
BMA House
Tavistock Square
London WC1H 9JP.

Osteopath

Osteopaths concentrate on treating back pain, and joint and muscle problems. However, they can also contribute to the treatment of various other medical problems, including the treatment of hyperactive children and menstrual problems.

DAY-TO-DAY WORK

Often people practise in a number of different places throughout the week, to reach a wider range of clients. Most osteopaths work in a conventional practice room, but some who have special expertise, e.g. in the problems of dancers or athletes, will work in dance studios or sports clubs. Some theatres have attached osteopaths who check performers regularly for signs of strain, so that possible damage can be prevented at an early stage.

Co-operation with colleagues in related subjects such as physiotherapy is often possible, and there is a growing trend for more communication with medical practitioners.

CAREER ROUTES AND TRAINING

Qualified doctors can become osteopaths by taking short additional courses. Those who are new to the area take a four to five year course which covers anatomy, physiology and pathology, as well as the specialist osteopathic manipulations of the body.

A broad general education with a scientific bias is required. Two science A-levels is usually the minimum requirement, although not all courses stick rigidly to this. A high proportion of students are re-training, with a view to starting a second career. These students are assessed on their prior learning and experience.

After qualification most students seek work as an assistant to a senior practitioner, before setting up their own practice.

For further information, write to:

British College of Naturopathy and Osteopathy
Frazer House
6 Netherall Gardens
London NW3 5RR.

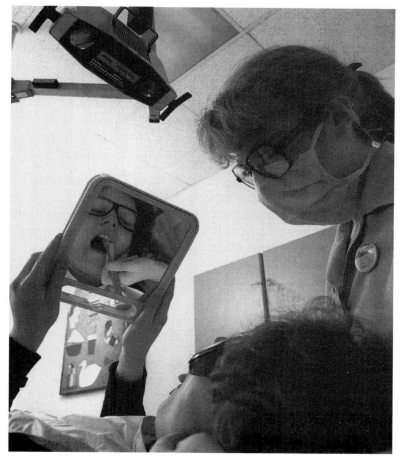

Figure 3.7   *A dentist at work*

Dentists

Dentists have an equally long training, and may work in hospitals or dental training schools as specialists. Most dentists, however, work in practice in the community, alone or in a group. Increasingly, dentists are working outside the National Health Service, seeing patients privately. Working hours are more regular than for doctors, though there may be a small amount of out of hours emergency work.

There are a number of jobs associated with dentistry, which require less training and qualifications. Dental technicians make dental appliances such as dentures and crowns; they do this in a workshop, supplying what dentists request. Dental therapists and hygienists carry out simple dental care and treatment such as cleaning and scaling teeth, and advise on dental health. Dental surgery assistants are the dentists' chairside helps.

Radiographers

Radiographers work in hospitals with X-rays, and can specialise in either diagnostic radiography (using techniques to help doctors diagnose broken bones and other conditions) or using radiation to treat patients with diseases such as cancer. This is called therapeutic radiography or radiotherapy.

Physiotherapists

Physiotherapists help sick, injured and disabled people to overcome movement problems and to be as physically independent as possible. They use a range of clinical skills, exercises, massage, heat and electrical treatment and hydrotherapy. They also teach people to avoid injury, e.g. the sort of back injuries you can get if you lift heavy objects wrongly. Besides working in the health service, physiotherapists can also work in private practice or for sports clubs etc.

Occupational therapists

Occupational therapists help patients of all ages to lead a more independent life at home and at work. They help people to find ways around day-to-day problems, and get them to improve their skills through activities which will get their muscles and joints working properly. They also advise on gadgets and alterations which may help people in their own homes, and encourage and enable them to enjoy creative activities. Occupational therapists mainly work in the health service, but some are employed by social services departments (see Fig. 3.5 page 92).

Opticians

Eye tests are carried out either by an optometrist, working in an optician's shop, or by a doctor who specialises in opthalmics. When you go to choose some new spectacles or contact lenses, a dispensing optician pro-

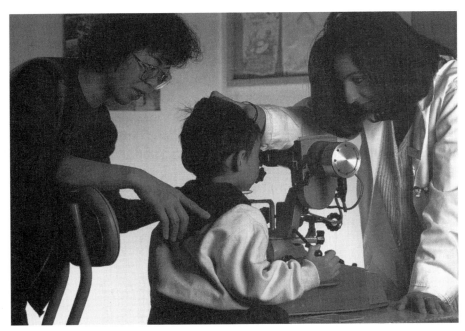

Figure 3.8   *An optician treats people of all ages*

vides these, working from the optometrist's prescription.

HOSPITAL NURSE

DAY-TO-DAY WORK

'The first step is to forget everything you thought you knew about hospitals, doctors and nurses.'

Many people see nursing as a series of practical procedures, such as dressing a wound or giving an injection. However, a professional nurse also needs to be able to observe and assess a particular case or situation, and decide what to do next. Choosing the right course of nursing action is more important than simply applying a set practical procedure.

CASE STUDY I

Maureen, a middle-aged woman, has just returned to her hospital bed after an operation on her gall bladder. Although she is naturally tired after the operation, she also feels in need of 'freshening-up'. A quick clean would give the ward sister an opportunity to check the operation wound and intravenous drip.

In the next ward lies a young man, Tony, who is on bed-rest because he is in traction with a broken leg. He can do most things for himself however, and feels that he is perfectly all right. The same ward sister is about to visit him. She is very aware of the dangers of prolonged bed-rest, such as blood-clots, respiratory infections and pressure sores.

How should the ward sister deal with each patient?

COMMENT

ⓘ The main priority for Maureen after her operation is rest. Although it's a good idea to change her position to prevent pressure sores occurring, and to help freshen her up, she will probably not appreciate the

ward sister taking an age to clean her inch by inch. She really needs to be left alone to rest as much as possible.

Tony on the other hand is probably bored! He needs encouragement to carry out what exercise he can, and to change position regularly to prevent the bed-rest dangers that might occur. The sister would spend much longer with him, and try to involve him in his own recovery programme as much as possible. She would explain what could happen if he doesn't move about, and get him motivated enough to carry out his own exercise programme without being prompted by her.

These two cases are typical of the variation between patients under a ward nurse's care. The *practical caring* skills of checking and monitoring recovery need to be combined with *social* and *communication* skills that the nurse will use to fully appreciate the client's own needs.

Mental health nurse

A mental health nurse deals with a wide range of conditions. While as many as one in three people suffer from some kind of mental health problem, only a small number are now admitted to hospital as part of their care programme. Most are cared for in the community. Some clients may have a serious and long-term mental illness, and need long-term care to enable them to live a life in the community. Others may reach a crisis point in their life when they are not able to cope; with the right nursing and medical care they may recover completely and not fall ill again.

DAY-TO-DAY WORK

With the increasing emphasis on community care, fewer mental health nurses work in hospital wards than before. In hospital, mental health nurses work in acute admission and

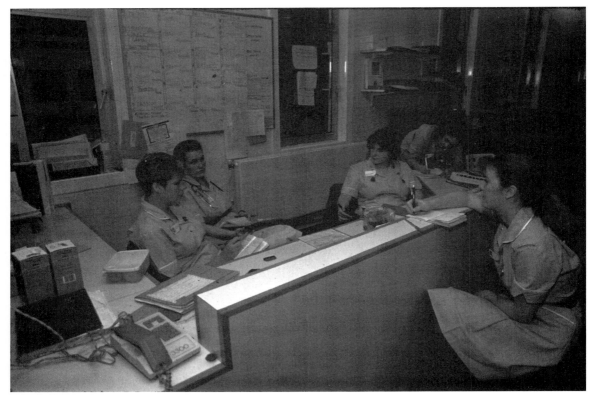

Figure 3.9   *Hospital nurses discussing their patients' care*

assessment wards. Out in the community, they may work in community-based projects such as half-way houses, group homes, or day centres.

One perception that exists is that mental health nurses have to deal with much violent behaviour. This is not the case, and in fact there may well be more violence in the Accident and Emergency department than in mental health units. However, one of the special skills of the mental health nurse is to spot the build-up of tension, and take the necessary action to defuse it.

Registered general nurses

CAREER ROUTES AND TRAINING

All training lasts for a minimum of three years before a nurse can be registered for practice, and takes place within a College of Nursing. Colleges look for a broad-based education, and ask for a minimum of five GCSEs or the equivalent, although some vocational qualifications are now also being accepted. All colleges are attached to a higher education institution, and those with two A levels or equivalent may well choose to follow a full nursing degree course.

All nurses complete a Common Foundation Programme for the first 18 months of the course, which provides an introduction to all aspects of modern nursing. The second half is taken up with one of the four branch programmes; adult nursing, mental health nursing, learning disability nursing, or children's nursing. Increasing amounts of time during the three years are spent on assignments, on hospital wards and in the community.

Once qualified, nurses are expected to keep up to date with the latest developments in clinical and professional practice. Many do this by adding further units to their existing qualification, arriving eventually at a full degree.

Career progression can follow several different ways. It is increasingly possible to specialise in a clinical area, moving from the ward hierarchy to become a clinical specialist in a particular area such as breast care.

Nurses can also move into a management role, either within a hospital setting, or in a health trust management team. Some become senior health service managers, helping to decide large policy issues affecting the care of local populations.

Those who find further study particularly rewarding can move into specialist research, helping to develop new approaches to improve care. Finally, nurse education is a good combination of continued client contact with developing new skills.

For further information, write to:

Careers Service
English National Board for Nursing
Midwifery and Health Visiting
PO Box 2EN
London W1A 2EN

Welsh National Board for Nursing
Midwifery and Health Visiting
13th Floor
Pearl Assurance House
Greyfriars Road
Cardiff CF1 3AG

The Nursing Advisor
Scottish Health Service Centre
Crewe Road South
Edinburgh EG4 2LF

The Recruitment Officer
National Board for Nursing
Midwifery and Health Visiting for
Northern Ireland
RAC House
79 Chichester Street
Belfast BT1 4JR.

Health visitor

A health visitor is a RGN who has taken a special course at a college of higher education or university. Most health visitors are attached to a particular GP, and are therefore responsible for the cases within that GP's practice, however widespread. Some are given defined areas though, and then work with many different GPs.

DAY-TO-DAY WORK

The health visitor decides who and when to visit, and takes referrals from others such as schools, health services and social workers. The pattern of visiting is based on the client's individual or family needs, and the health visitor will visit without necessarily being asked to call.

Many of the skills needed by health visitors are social skills, such as motivating individuals to change their diet or exercise pattern. They also need to be able to advise clients on issues such as when and whether to immunise young babies, and provide support in times of stress. Practical caring skills are also needed, for instance, when testing a baby's hearing.

A major focus is on health education and primary prevention, i.e. taking action before a disease or disability has taken hold; for instance, encouraging immunisation for diseases such as measles, rubella and polio; alternatively, giving advice and help to parents, children and elderly people on how to make their homes more safe, and reduce the risk of a home accident.

For further information, see nursing addresses on page 105.

District nurse

The district nurse is a qualified RGN, who has undertaken further training in a university. The aim is to gain specialised skills enabling the DN to care for clients outside the hospital setting, and also to arrange financial and social help for them if necessary.

DAY-TO-DAY WORK

The district nurse is a team leader in the primary health care team, delegating work to newly qualified nurses, nursing auxiliaries or care assistants. This level of responsibility is similar to a ward sister delegating work to the ward nurses.

Nearly all DNs are attached to a particular GP, and will look after patients referred to them by that GP. Some referrals also come directly from a hospital liaison sister. However, most of a DN's time is spent in the home of the client; their level of responsibility and also their independence is therefore very high.

It is important for the DN to communicate effectively with the client, as much of the role consists of secondary prevention, or preventing an illness or disability getting out of control. This might for example mean encouraging a client with dental problems to seek dental treatment. DNs also give care and support for rehabilitation, helping a client recover from a previous mental or physical illness. For instance, the DN might visit and support a woman who has had a mastectomy, helping her to deal with her feelings and prevent depression.

The district nurse will also work with the client's relatives or other carers to explain practical help or care that they can give. A frequent example might be showing safe lifting techniques to other carers. The DN is responsible for client care even when not with their patient, and in this way can try to ensure continuity of care wherever possible.

For further information, see nursing addresses on page 105.

Practice nurse

Both the Community Care Act 1990 and the change in funding arrangements for many GPs have had a great effect on the role of nurses working in the community. Many more GP practices now employ practice nurses, to support their work in health promotion and prevention.

DAY-TO-DAY WORK

Much of the day-to-day work consists of some, though hardly ever all, of the following:

- basic treatments such as ear syringing and treating minor injuries, vaccination and immunisation programmes
- screening programmes, such as cervical smear testing and Well Woman clinics
- providing advice on stopping smoking, weight reduction, retirement
- monitoring health of those with chronic illnesses such as diabetes or asthma
- helping with ante- and post-natal care, and family planning
- providing information and advice on services available to clients
- administration such as updating client records.

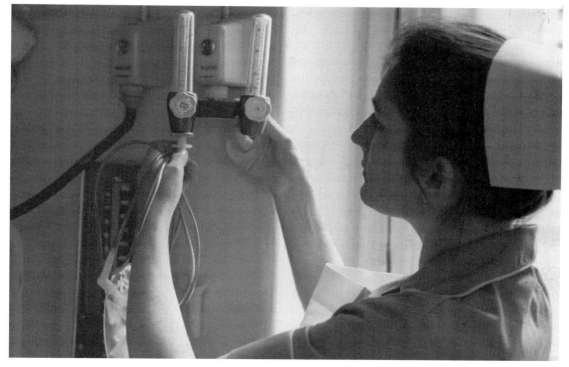

Figure 3.10   *There are many different kinds of nurse, and nursing care*

Midwife

Midwives either work in hospitals or in the community. Their practical skills involve caring for pregnant women, delivering their babies and supporting parents in caring for new-born babies at post-natal clinics and check-ups. For a normal birth, the midwife will be in charge, but a doctor will be required for a breech birth, Caesarean section or if complications ensue. They also need to be aware of social and cultural factors affecting the families they work with and the maternity care that is provided.

DAY-TO-DAY WORK

'Midwifery is as much about supporting women and their partners as the birth of their baby. My involvement can start even before a woman is pregnant, by providing pre-conception advice. I can then continue to support her from initial confirmation of pregnancy to the birth of her baby, and up to twenty-eight days afterwards.'

Practising midwife, 13 years experience

Much of the day-to-day work involves supervising and examining pregnant women, both in hospital wards and, increasingly, in the home. The midwife needs to be able to make decisions about what care is appropriate, and know when to involve other health professionals if something unexpected or untoward happens.

The central role of midwives is to assist

with the delivery of babies, and take a very active role in straightforward births. Moreover, they need to be able to cope in an emergency, and be familiar with the range of drugs and other treatments that might be used. Midwives also need to know what steps to take if a baby has a low birth-weight, or is ill at birth.

Midwives also provide care during pregnancy to women in the community, again working as part of a health care team with GPs, obstetricians and health visitors. Often this involves running parent education groups, where the midwife can get to know the prospective parents, and give advice and information to help increase their confidence. They keep contact with mothers after the birth, providing close care and support for another 28 days, and inviting them back to parental groups to share their experience with others.

As mothers become more confident, and expect to play a greater role in their own childbirth, so the midwife's role is becoming more demanding. The need to give day-to-day advice and support is just as important as the practical caring skills needed at the time of childbirth and immediately after.

CAREER ROUTES AND TRAINING

Midwives can follow a specialist course at a College of Midwifery and/or Nursing, where courses last for at least three years. Minimum requirements are five GCSEs or equivalent, to include English Language and a science subject. Many people however train first as a registered general nurse (RGN), and then do a post-graduate midwifery course for another 18 months.

Like nurses, all midwives then have responsibility to continue their own professional development. In particular this means they must be able to show that they have updated their knowledge by doing further training every five years.

Many go further in their careers by taking specialist training, in order to be able to advise on family planning for instance, or carry out intensive care of new-born babies. Others take advanced diploma and degree courses, either simply for greater knowledge and understanding, or to move towards teaching or research.

For further information, see nursing addresses on page 105.

SOCIAL CARERS

Social worker

DAY-TO-DAY WORK

Most social workers work within a geographical area, and liaise with many primary health care teams in that area. Some are however attached to General Practices, in the same way as nurses. In addition, social workers work in many different settings such as hospitals, residential homes, children's homes and with voluntary agencies such as the NSPCC.

In some areas social workers concentrate either on a particular client group, such as disabled people, or upon different phases of work, such as local community development schemes.

The main client groups are elderly people, families in which there are neglected or abused children, or children whose behaviour is beyond control. Social workers also work with offenders, disabled people, and emotionally distressed people. With the emphasis on community care, there is an increased amount of work with elderly people who might previously have lived in hospitals or residential homes.

The main social role is to provide advice and support, and practical help for those individuals and families who have severe social problems. There is also however a great deal of administration and paperwork to be done. There are records for each client to keep, and much dealing with other agencies. Social workers may also become involved in court cases and legal procedures.

Social work can be emotionally demanding; some clients can be very uncooperative and even hostile, and there may be no real solution to long-term problems. It can be difficult to appreciate and understand clients' problems without becoming personally involved, or to carry on trying to help aggressive or unco-operative clients. On top of this, hours are often irregular, as social problems need to be dealt with at any time.

CAREER ROUTES AND TRAINING

Training for social work and social care is run by the Central Council for Education and Training in Social Work (CCETSW). The main qualification is a Diploma in Social Work, which is gained after a two year programme run jointly by educational institutions and social work agencies. Some courses are college-based, some employment-based, and some offer a combination of both. All new students under the age of 21 must have two A levels or the equivalent (including Advanced GNVQ Health and Social Care).

The three main routes for social workers are within local authority social services departments, local education authorities, and the probation service. Within social services, social workers can also work for county councils, overseeing provision of care at a wider regional level.

For further information, write to CCETSW Information Service at:

Derbyshire House
St Chad's Street
London WC1H 8AD

78–80 George Street
Edinburgh EG2 3BU

6 Malone Road
Belfast BT9 5BN

West Wing
2nd Floor
Southgate House
Wood Street
Cardiff CF1 1EW

Counsellor

Counselling has been described as the art of listening constructively. Most counsellors say that they are non-directive, i.e. their purpose is not to influence their clients to act in a particular way, but to help them explore their situation and the options open to them, and then make their own decisions.

Counselling is considered appropriate for clients dealing with difficult life situations and emotional problems, but not people with severe mental illness. It is undertaken by many different practitioners, both in the course of practising other disciplines, and as a practice on its own. For those wanting to counsel as a profession in itself, there are many training courses available, through universities, private training courses, or courses run by groups with one particular approach or doctrine.

DAY-TO-DAY WORK

Counselling takes place in many different settings; within the NHS and social services, as part of the work of voluntary organisations such as Cruse, Relate and the Samaritans, and in private practice.

The day-to-day working conditions vary a great deal according to the local priorities placed upon the counselling service.

Counsellors in private practice need to decide where they should hold sessions, bear-

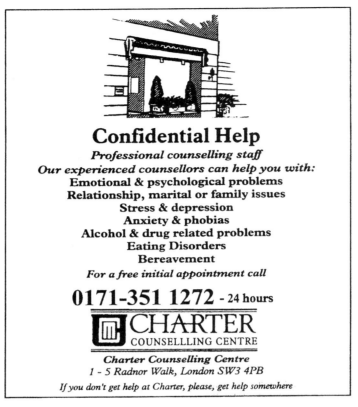

Confidential Help

Professional counselling staff
Our experienced counsellors can help you with:
Emotional & psychological problems
Relationship, marital or family issues
Stress & depression
Anxiety & phobias
Alcohol & drug related problems
Eating Disorders
Bereavement

For a free initial appointment call

0171-351 1272 - 24 hours

CHARTER
COUNSELLLING CENTRE

Charter Counselling Centre
1 - 5 Radnor Walk, London SW3 4PB
If you don't get help at Charter, please, get help somewhere

Figure 3.11   *Counselling can play a vital role in social care*

ing in mind their own need for privacy and that of the client for confidentiality. Working at home has some advantages, such as convenience and informality, but client confidentiality may be difficult to maintain. Many counsellors feel that hiring a room in a professional practice suite is better.

Counselling is not a well-paid profession, and in fact many practitioners start off with unpaid work in the voluntary sector, in order to gain professional experience.

CAREER ROUTES AND TRAINING

Counselling is a popular choice for a second career. This is because people are seldom mature enough on leaving school or university. Entry to training courses is usually with a degree, although by no means all entrants have one. Most important is a selection interview, where those able to contribute to a group process are looked for.

Courses are usually about two years long leading to a diploma, or one year leading to a certificate. Short courses are also available from many of the same sources mentioned above.

Most counsellors take part in regular in-service training, and to start with, will have a supervisor in the form of a senior counsellor. Later the individual will move on to become a supervisor himself. This ensures that the practitioner continues to learn throughout their career, and maintains professional skills at the highest standard. It also provides emotional support by giving an opportunity for discussion with an experienced colleague in a regular and structured way. The British Association for Counsellors has a category of Accredited Counsellors who have followed this route.

For further information, write to:

The British Association for Counselling
37A Sheep Street
Rugby CV21 3BX.

Care assistant

DAY-TO-DAY WORK

Care assistants work in day centres, residential homes, nursing homes and hospitals. On hospital wards they carry out many of the practical caring tasks that were previously carried out by enrolled nurses. Their practical work involves providing care and help with everyday living needs, such as getting about, dressing, bathing, eating and recreation.

Like other carers, social skills are also a necessary part of the care assistant's role. They have to be sensitive to the frustrations of people who have lost much independence and encourage them to do as much as possible for themselves (even when it would be quicker to do things for them).

Domiciliary care assistants help clients, mainly elderly people, in their own home. Their clients are basically well, but need help with the same everyday tasks mentioned above.

Those who visit clients in their own homes usually work fairly regular hours. Residential care assistant work necessarily involves 'unsocial' hours, including evenings and weekends.

CAREER ROUTES AND TRAINING

Care assistants have traditionally been unqualified, and have gained on-the-job training and experience. NVQs have now been developed at Levels 2 and 3 so that care assistants can show their competence and gain a recognised qualification.

Here are some of the things that those who have recently achieved NVQ awards said it meant to them:

- greater awareness of clients' needs and rights, especially emotional, social and cultural needs
- more able to give individual care to clients
- being better informed, more assertive and confident, and more able to challenge inadequate practice

SUPPORT SERVICES

Clinic assistant/manager

In the past, many very successful GP practices have been built on common sense and high standards of professional practice. The pattern now however is for increasing numbers of practitioners to work together in group practices representing a wide range of professional skills. With a clinic manager in place, the many services and facilities that the practitioners need are professionally provided, so that each practitioner is able to concentrate on the business of looking after their clients.

DAY-TO-DAY WORK

Essentially the business side can be seen as organising the space available, letting some areas perhaps to those working outside the practice, such as physiotherapists or counsellors. In addition, book-keeping and accountancy, building management, hotel and conference management and personnel management skills could all be called for.

CAREER ROUTES AND TRAINING

There are a number of ways of becoming a clinic manager. Obviously an interest in the work of the practitioners and a knowledge of what they offer to clients is necessary, although it does not have to be a detailed knowledge.

The experience of working as a receptionist and moving up the career ladder as opportunities arise, can lead to a more responsible position within a large group practice.

Administrative staff

These are the people who see that everything runs efficiently. This means, for example, checking that money is spent correctly, ordering supplies, making sure that record systems work, taking on and training staff etc. There are general managers, personnel managers, accountants, supplies officers, catering managers, domestic superintendents, computer staff, and many others.

Clerical staff

These do the day-to-day paper work. There are secretaries and receptionists, computer operators and medical records officers, amongst others.

Practical task are carried out by maintenance staff, cooks and catering assistants, laundry assistants, porters, and many other vital members of the team.

We have seen that there are very many different jobs at several different levels, in the health and social care services. Not surprisingly, people arrive at these jobs via many different routes.

These are only a few examples of the diverse backgrounds of health and social care workers!

How clear a view does the general public

CASE STUDY 2

Mary was not very interested in school work, and left with no qualifications. She got a job as a dentist's chairside assistant. Mary did this for several years, and found she enjoyed the contact with people in a health care setting. She decided to go back to college to study for some GCSEs. Having successfully completed these, she applied to a hospital and was accepted for training as a nurse. She is now a qualified registered general nurse (RGN), working happily in a busy hospital ward.

Graham graduated in history at university. He had done a certain amount of voluntary work with young people, and after obtaining his degree, went to work in a children's home as a child care assistant for a couple of years. He then applied to a college to train as a social worker. After qualification, Graham obtained a post as a social worker in a local authority department. While there, he took further part-time training to specialise in working with people with psychiatric problems, and his next post was as a social worker in a psychiatric hospital. He is still employed in the health service, but has moved to a more managerial position, involved with the purchasing by his local authority of care services, having studied in his own time to gain a management qualification.

Jane trained as a cook when she left school, and worked in restaurants and pubs, before securing a job in a residential home for old people. She became very interested in care work, and began to help out in this capacity. Showing aptitude for it, after some time she was offered the opportunity to go on a day-release training course. Now, some years later, and having obtained further qualifications and experience, she is herself the manager of a private residential home for people with disabilities.

---

have of what health and social care workers actually do? Try the following activity.

Activity 9

1 Over the next week, see how many news stories you can find in the local or national newspapers, or on the television news, which mention the involvement of a social worker in the events described. Note down the main facts of the cases.

2 How much can you find out from this about what the social worker actually did in the situation? Make a list of the comments that are made that are a) critical, b) approving, of how the social worker is said to have acted.

3 In your group, draw on what you have learned about the job of social workers, to discuss what you think might have happened that was not reported in the news stories. How do you think the social workers concerned feel about what happened? Imagine you are some of the other people involved in the events. What do you think they feel about what has happened? Does their anger or frustration mean that the social workers could have acted differently? If so, what prevented their doing so?

4 You may feel that it is not possible to answer these questions from what you read or hear in the news. Perhaps your tutor might arrange for a social worker to come and talk to you about their experiences in similar situations.

You could choose another job, perhaps that of a health care worker, and repeat the above exercise.

Activity 10

Rates of pay change within health and caring occupations from year to year, but some professions are clearly better paid than others.

Discuss within groups what levels of pay the roles above might receive. How would you go about finding out what actual levels of pay are? See how your list compares with the reality.

COMMENT

Job advertisements often, though not always, specify a range of pay (salary scale) for a particular job. For further details on pay for health service professions, write to:

Health Service Careers
PO Box 204
London SE99 7UW

SUMMARY

- Everyone needs care and support from other people at certain times.
- Some people have particular needs because of disability, illness, or social circumstances.
- The state takes responsibility for much health and social care provision.
- A state with many statutory services is called a welfare state.
- Much care is still given within the family or by other informal means.
- Voluntary organisations play an important part in providing care.
- The National Health Service was set up in 1948. It provides hospitals and community health services.
- The Department of Social Security administers financial help.
- Social service departments are local authority departments with responsibility for personal social services.
- The NHS and Community Care Act 1990 was an important milestone. It placed a lot of emphasis on supporting people in their own homes wherever possible.
- Social service departments make a variety of provision including residential and community care.
- Groups needing particular support are children, adolescents, mentally and physically handicapped people and elderly people.
- Easy access to the available services is essential.
- Clients have a right to be treated with dignity, to be given choice, and to be enabled to remain as independent as possible.

- Clients have a right not to be discriminated against and to be guaranteed confidentiality.
- Many different jobs exist within health and social care services. Training, responsibilities and career paths vary considerably.

DEFINITIONS

Advocate someone who speaks or acts on behalf of a person not able to act for himself.

Bereavement loss of someone or something valued, usually referring to loss by death.

Client someone who uses a service provided.

Community care care which aims to help people to live as independently as possible, in their own homes.

Culture the values, attitudes and customs shared by a group of people, and handed on by them.

Disability/handicap a physical or mental condition that prevents a person from doing something.

Domiciliary care care that is given by care assistants employed to work in clients' own homes.

Extended family a social unit consisting of not only a couple and their children, but other relatives, e.g. aunts, uncles, grandparents.

Health services services to promote health and well-being and to prevent and treat ill-health.

Informal carers people who voluntarily help to look after others, not as a paid job; usually family, friends or neighbours.

Learning disability/difficulty a condition acquired before, at, or soon after birth, that affects a person's development and ability to learn the ordinary skills of daily living.

Mobility ability to move freely and independently from place to place.

Primary care care, often preventative, delivered in the community.

Professional carers people who are trained, qualified and paid to give care.

Secondary care care, often curative, provided in hospital situations.

Social services services provided by the community to help those in need.

Social services department a local authority department which employs social workers to provide mainly personal social services.

Tertiary care care provided through long-term rehabilitation.

Voluntary organisation an association or society, usually a nonprofit-making charity, that has been created by its members, not by the state.

Welfare state provision by the government of a system of social services; these are called statutory services.

4

COMMUNICATION AND INTERPERSONAL RELATIONSHIPS

AIMS AND OBJECTIVES

The aim of this chapter is to help you to understand the importance of effective communication and good interpersonal relationships in health and social care. You need to develop your own communication skills first of all, and the activities will help you practice this skill.

At the end of this chapter, you should have:

- developed your own communication skills

- understood the effects of discrimination against others

- identified aspects of communication between clients and carers in health and social care settings

Developing communication skills

COMMUNICATION BETWEEN GROUPS, FAMILIES AND INDIVIDUALS

In this section we are going to look more closely at what happens when people interact so that we can be more aware of our effect on any encounter we find ourselves in. This applies particularly to caring relationships as well as more generally to other relationships with individuals or groups; such as friendships, working relationships, being a member of a team, relationships with teachers, students and many more.

Activity 1

 Take some paper and list as many things as you can think of that happen in conversation and social interaction. Do not worry if they seem obvious, it is the obvious which is often missed!

COMMENT

Here are some of the things you may have included:

1 Sharing ideas and opinions as well as thoughts and feelings.

2 Attempting to understand the difference between people.

3 Trying to find out about yourself by finding how others 'tick'.

4 Hoping to be accepted by another person or as a member of a group.

5 Trying to prove to yourself and others that you are 'good enough', or that you have special talents and a personality which you would like others to see: these are the parts of yourself that you value.

6 Hoping that others do not see some of the parts of yourself which you do not like, about which you might feel embarrassed or ashamed, or that if they do, that they will not dislike you.

7 Expressing strong feelings such as anger or sorrow.

There are many more, but from your own list and the list above it is evident that a common factor in communication is the expression of need and the meeting of need. As you can see from the list of definitions at the end of this chapter, self-esteem is described as a way of feeling good about yourself. Other people can help us to feel good about ourselves, so this is an important aspect of conversation.

DEVELOPMENT OF SELF

Doing Activity 1 involves learning about yourself and relationships with other people. Sometimes this means facing personal difficulties and as a result, feeling upset and seeing the activity as a waste of time. Despite the difficulties involved, many people find this process, known as *self development*, worthwhile and that it helps them form bet-

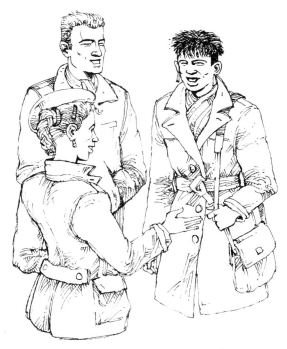

Figure 4.1 *Social interaction is an essential part of human life*

ter relationships with themselves and others. Being able to care for others effectively involves being able to know about and care for yourself.

An example of self development: you might know a man who always blames other people for everything that goes wrong in his life. Imagine meeting him in a couple of years time to find that he was able to tell you that he used to blame everybody because he felt a total failure. Now, he tells you, he has a job and a girlfriend and although he still loses his temper from time to time he is able to see that it is caused by his own frustration rather than other people some of whom were in fact doing their best to help him.

Self development means we become more aware of the effect we have on others as well as the other way around. Although this sometimes means facing some unlikeable parts of ourselves, such as strong feelings of hurt, anger and fear, we usually end up feeling better about ourselves and others. Many people do not talk about these parts of themselves because they fear others would not like them anymore. If you actually try it, you will probably find that people end up liking you more for your courage, honesty and straightforwardness. The key to all of this is good communication, and we will later see how good communication can help self development while bad communication hinders it.

PERSONAL PREFERENCES AND BELIEFS

We all have different preferences and beliefs, although it is sometimes hard to accept this. It usually seems easier to get on with someone who is similar to us. They may have similar interests, be of a similar age or have the same political or religious beliefs. When faced with someone who is very different from us, it can be more of a challenge to feel at ease with them. Again, good communication can help us overcome these barriers and find the real person underneath the differences on the surface. Feelings of sadness, joy, pain and anger are in everybody, no matter what they believe.

DEVELOPMENT OF GROUPS AND FAMILIES

Just as individuals can develop and become more aware of themselves in relation to others, so too can groups and families. Think for a moment about your study group and how it has changed since the first time together. If you did not know each other

beforehand you might have found the first few meetings rather uncomfortable until you got to know people. By looking at groups, we can see that some groups work better than others; e.g. a group which is split between clever/not so clever, tall/short, smoking/non smoking, or outgoing/shy is not likely to work well. That sort of group will have winners and losers. On the other hand a group (including a family) that can understand and put up with differences, is likely to be a better place for all the group members. The positive change of a group that does not work well for everybody, to one that does, is part of group development and made possible with good communication skills as we will see later in this chapter.

LISTENING AND RESPONDING SKILLS

Scenario

Imagine you come home to find a friend, Jane, waiting for you, wanting to talk. Although you wanted to catch up with some work before going out, you see how upset she is and invite her in. She sits down and starts to cry. After a while you find out that she has split up from her boyfriend and feels really sad. You already know that this is not the first time this has happened and is beginning to become a pattern. You feel like telling her to be more selective in her choice of boyfriend, but remember that other friends have told her this before and the advice has made little difference. You feel worried and a bit annoyed because she repeats her mistakes and has become less fun to be with.

Activity 2

 Think for a moment about what is useful to you when you are upset.

Take a blank piece of paper and make two columns. Head the first one 'caring' and the second 'uncaring'.

COMMENT

Perhaps your list included some of the following (remember, there is no right or wrong here; my list includes what most people find caring when they are upset):

Caring: warmth, gentle tone of voice, listening, space, relaxed posture, eye contact, accepting attitude, understanding.

Uncaring: judging, hurrying, tense posture, giving advice, offering solutions rather than being understanding.

Activity 3

 Suppose, in the scenario above, your friend starts by saying:

'John just told me he doesn't want to go out with me any more, he says I'm too possessive and he can't stand my jealousy.'

Think for a moment how you might react. What could you say that would be helpful? Read the following statements and say which seem helpful and which seem unhelpful:

1 'Couldn't you try to be less possessive?'
2 Sitting leaning forward.
3 'You must be really upset.'
4 'Do you think he is going out with someone else?'
5 Sitting in a relaxed way with arms on your lap while looking directly at Jane.

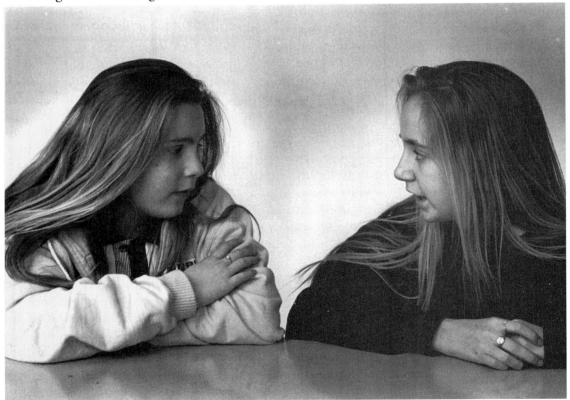

Figure 4.2   *Do you have a friend in whom you could confide if you needed help?*

6 Just not saying anything for a little while.

7 'I'm sure you'll find someone else soon.'

8 Sitting with arms folded and looking away.

9 'That must have been a real shock.'

10 'Perhaps you could say a little more about what happened.'

COMMENT

These are my answers but please remember there are no hard and fast rules to helpful communication, just guidelines:

1 uncaring: seems quite judgemental and does not take Jane's feelings into account. Perhaps well intended and may be true, but fails to understand Jane from her own point of view.

2 uncaring: inappropriate non-verbal behaviour, could seem threatening, does not give feeling of space.

3 caring: shows you are hearing Jane's feelings and not just what she says. Demonstrates that you are trying to understand how she feels from her own point of view.

4 uncaring: this response might at best be a good guess, but fails to connect to how Jane feels and may well upset her more.

5 caring: a relaxed posture conveys a willingness to give time and space. Eye contact helps to form a 'bridge' between people.

6 caring: a short silence, which sometimes may seem awkward, is often very welcome to someone who is upset as it allows them time to gather their thoughts and helps them not to feel rushed.

7 uncaring: although well meant this could produce the opposite effect since it conveys a message that you might rather not hear about how sad and upset Jane is.

8 uncaring: this non verbal message suggests that you are shutting Jane out with your arms and keeping her away by not engaging eye contact.

9 caring: this shows you have understood how Jane feels and that you are willing to be with her while she experiences difficult and painful feelings.

10 caring: this is an open question which invites Jane to say more if she wants to so that she can explore issues and feelings around her break-up. It is important that this choice is left to her. A closed question such as; 'Tell me what happened,' is more like a demand and could seem threatening to Jane.

Scenario

You are doing some voluntary work for the elderly in a residential home and you are assigned to help a man in his eighties called Pablo who is recovering from a stroke (which can affect movement and memory as well as producing a general feeling of confusion and sometimes despair).

Your task is further complicated by the fact that Pablo seems to prefer to speak in Portuguese. He spent the first twenty eight years of his life in Brazil before moving to England with his wife, a nurse, who died ten years ago.

Imagine you are in the dining room with Pablo having a cup of tea and are struggling to understand his story about his family who lived in great poverty. He has told you that he feels bad that he has left them behind and has not been back to see them, although he has sent them money on a regular basis. His attention frequently wanders and he is often quite demanding of you, asking for things to be done for him all the time. He often shouts angrily and you are wondering if someone else could take over from you, but you realise that he would probably be the same with anyone so you carry on.

Activity 4

 In groups of three, discuss and record your group's main views on the following:

1 What is Pablo feeling at the moment?
2 What needs is he indirectly 'asking' you to meet?
3 What factors make it difficult for Pablo to express his needs?
4 How do you know what these needs are if he does not tell you?
5 What can you do to:
   a identify Pablo's needs?
   b help Pablo express his needs?
   c meet Pablo's needs?
6 Are there any limits on **5 a**, **b**, and **c**? If so, what are they and how can you work within those limits to help Pablo?

COMMENT

 The following are examples of possible answers:

1 Pablo could be feeling confused, helpless, angry and guilty.
2 He appears to be 'asking' you to understand him and put up with him. Perhaps one message is: 'I don't like myself very much at the moment, and I am trying to make you dislike me as well to prove I am right.' If you manage to hear this hidden message and then continue to try to accept and be warm to him then there is a chance he will begin to feel a little bit better about himself.
3 The following factors make it difficult for Pablo to express his needs:
   a Pablo's age and background might make him feel very different from you. He might find it difficult to believe that you could understand him. His illness has made him prefer to use his mother tongue which you probably do not speak.

   b His physical disabilities. His limited movement due to the effects of stroke make it difficult for him to use non-verbal messages effectively. This would add to his feeling of helplessness.
   c His mental disabilities. The effects of a stroke can alter personality in unpredictable ways, making a person unable to know what they might need, never mind express those needs.
   d The effect of any medication Pablo might be taking.
4 You will not necessarily understand all Pablo's needs, but will get a feel for them through the use of empathy (see definition of terms, pages 142–144). By recognising certain universal needs you will be able to fill in the gaps where Pablo cannot express himself. One way of doing this is to look at how he is making you feel. It is quite likely that he is making you feel like he feels; you can then use this as a guide to help him.
5 **a** You will be able to hear Pablo's spoken or 'hidden' messages if you are reflectively listening (see page 26). If you can hear these 'needs messages' then you will be able to identify them.
   b By reflectively listening and helping Pablo identify and clarify what he needs you will help him express his needs. For example commenting, 'You seem worried about your relatives', may help him to focus more clearly on how he is feeling at the moment and indicates that you have heard and understood him.
   c By being there and listening you are already meeting some of Pablo's needs. There are some other more practical needs (such as helping him write to his family, or arranging for him to be more comfortable), which you can meet once you have identified them.
6 There are obviously going to be limits on the

amount of care you can offer Pablo. There are some aspects of his situation which will not improve much and all you can do is to help him adjust to his level of disability. By being with a lonely and confused old man in a helpful way, by reflectively listening and trying to understand him from his own point of view you will be meeting some of his needs and helping him to express his own needs. You will be providing a quality of interpersonal relationship which will make him feel better about himself.

HOW DO WE COMMUNICATE?

Let us now look more closely at what happens in communication. I am going to break down communication and responding into a number of parts, some of which you will be more or less aware of at any one time.

Facial expression

Our faces communicate a great deal about how we are feeling. The muscles behind the skin can arrange the face to produce a huge range of expressions. These expressions carry meanings which vary in different cultures. Anger, hope, rage, love, joy, sorrow, warmth, concern, superiority, inferiority, fear and panic are some of the feelings that a facial expression can communicate.

Body language and posture

We communicate with our bodies all the time, sometimes without being aware of it. Body language and posture refer to the way we move our hands, arms, legs and feet as well as the way we hold our head. When we talk we often use our hands to make a point. There is a whole language (apart from sign-ing) in hand movements which vary considerably in their meaning according to where you are: a pointed finger might draw attention to a particular point in one culture and be an obscene gesture in another; a 'V' sign can be 'victory' or something much ruder depending on which way round the hand is held. (The obscene 'V' sign is said to originate from the time when archers had their arrow-holding fingers removed as a punishment. The original 'V' sign was therefore a taunt, meaning: 'Look what I have got and you have not.' The meaning has changed with time.)

A handshake can be firm and friendly, or harsh and aggressive. Someone who offers their hand palm down may be putting you down (by having to respond palm up you could be seen to be saying: 'Look I have nothing.'). All these examples have to be taken in context; e.g. a tilted head can mean: 'Go on, I am listening.' In another context it can mean: 'Do I have to put up with this drivel for much longer!' Eye contact and facial expression are part of the total message.

Try observing the way people walk. I will give three examples and suggested interpretations: see Fig. 4.3.

1 Head held high, back straight, long strides with eyes looking ahead – this seems to suggest confidence and certainty of purpose.
2 As 1 above but with a swaying side to side motion, with a slight lean backwards (this is perhaps more of a male characteristic in our culture) – this is a 'swagger', suggesting arrogance and perhaps compensating for feelings of inferiority.
3 Looking down, dragging the feet, sometimes stopping, walking with slow limp movements – this person seems to be rather sad or depressed.

These examples may seem rather obvious,

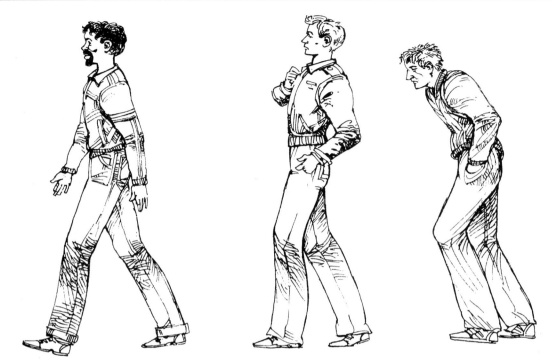

Figure 4.3   *Body language can indicate a mood or even a person's character*

but it is the obvious which we so often miss because we see it all the time. By thinking about what we do with our bodies and what that might mean, we start to see people in a different way. Try it for yourself:

Activity 5

This is a game of charades, but instead of a film, book or play you are to try to act the following (you can extend the list). The remainder of your group is to guess what you are saying with your body.

- I am bored
- I am too beautiful to be around here
- I am really fed up
- I am angry at being stood up
- I am lonely and sad
- I am really important
- I am tough

When you do this, try to identify the aspects of body language which say the most and feed them back to the 'actor'. This way you will be able to identify what gestures or postures mean. If you are observant the next time you are in a public place and learn to 'read' body language you will be surprised at how much you will learn about interpersonal relationships.

Non-verbal messages

These can be broken down into parts:

1 *Eyes:* amount of contact, nervous blinking, staring, narrowing or widening of eyes, winking, smiling eyes, cross eyes, tearful eyes.
2 *Face:* a large number of expressions can be produced to indicate different emotions, (see above, p. 121).

Activity 6

 To do this activity you need to find a partner with whom you are going to have a 'non-verbal conversation'.

You will need a chair to sit on and your partner should stand about one metre away.

In this 'conversation', imagine that you are on holiday in China and are trying to order a meal in a local restaurant (if you speak Chinese then please think of somewhere else!). You can play the tourist and your partner the waiter/waitress. The menu is written in Chinese and there is no display of food.

You can do anything except speak, get out of the chair, or touch your partner. You will need to remember that your partner comes from a different culture to you and you cannot assume that he or she eats the same food as you do, but remember that you are very hungry and must find something to eat.

Facial expression as well as the use of the hands, arms and shoulders can probably express more than you expect. As you communicate, try to notice how you express understanding, perhaps with a nod or a smile. This understanding will then enable your partner to know that the message has been communicated, who will be confident in using the same non-verbal signals again. If, on the other hand, your message has not been understood, then note the way your partner lets you know this, perhaps with a shake of the head or a frown.

When you think you have successfully ordered a meal you can ask (with words) what you would have been served with. Was it what you wanted? If it was, how do you feel? How would you feel if it was something you could not bring yourself to eat even if you are really hungry? Annoyed or perhaps let down?

Now change places and try the other way around.

After a while (about ten or fifteen minutes) you may notice the 'non-verbal conversation' become easier; why is this?

COMMENT

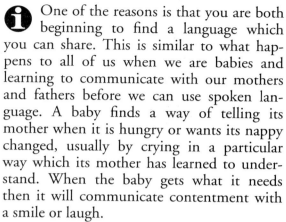 One of the reasons is that you are both beginning to find a language which you can share. This is similar to what happens to all of us when we are babies and learning to communicate with our mothers and fathers before we can use spoken language. A baby finds a way of telling its mother when it is hungry or wants its nappy changed, usually by crying in a particular way which its mother has learned to understand. When the baby gets what it needs then it will communicate contentment with a smile or laugh.

Notice here how the mother has to learn a language as well as the baby in a *two way learning process*. There are two important points which I want to raise about this exercise in 'non-verbal conversation':

Communication is two-way. It involves trying to understand as well as trying to say or express something.

When we communicate with someone it is important to note that the effort to understand is just as important as the effort to communicate. It is not very useful to go abroad and start ordering a meal in a restaurant without checking what the waiter/waitress can understand. What you say to him or her will depend on what you know will be understood. If for example you find out that he or she cannot speak a word of English (and assuming that you do not speak the local language) then you will probably have to do something like the exercise above. Even if you think you know a language well, it does not follow that you will be understood or will be able to understand how someone really feels.

To illustrate this, think how you may sometimes have felt misunderstood by parents or teachers or anyone who has a different outlook from your own. Remember how hard it can be to get someone to see things from your point of view when they are set on making you agree with them.

Even a road sign has an element of a two-way communication about it. The designer has to consider carefully the people looking at the sign and what it might be mistaken for, so he or she can produce a message that is not confusing.

Being understood makes us feel better about ourselves.

When we communicate and are understood, what happens? Think back to your role-play in the restaurant: smiles, nods and smiling eyes perhaps? When we are understood we sense that someone knows something we want them to know and that makes us feel we can get what we need from another person. This understanding can be broken down into two parts:

1 The factual part of understanding: e.g. 'I like fried fish,' which is important, because without communicating that part you would not get the meal you expected. For many people this seems the most important part of the communication.

2 Being understood can make us feel accepted and good. Why is this? When we know we are understood we feel a bridge has been built up between us and another person and we feel less alone. However bad things are, being understood makes us feel a bit better.

Imagine you are a little baby. You feel hungry, wet and too hot. You cry loudly and no one comes to make things better. Because you cannot understand that mum is on the phone you get angry and perhaps frightened that you will never be made comfortable. So you cry louder and more angrily.

Mum eventually gets the message and says to her friend that she has to go, her baby is too upset to leave any longer.

Mum comes over to you and picks you up. At first you are angry with her for abandoning you and you refuse to be fed, but eventually she seems to accept your rage and you gratefully accept her comforting food. At last you feel that you are understood which enables you to take the food, which you could not until your anger was understood and accepted.

Sensory contact

This covers physical contact of any kind, such as touching, holding or attending to personal needs such as combing hair. Sensory contact can have a number of meanings depending on the situation and it is very important that we are clear about these different meanings.

For example, holding the hand of an elderly resident in a care situation when she is crying over her lost cat may have a very different meaning from the same action between a man and woman on their first outing together. The intention of the first action is primarily to comfort, while the intention of the second action *may* be to signal the message 'I want to get closer to you'. Of course it could have the same meaning as with the old lady, this depends on the circumstances. The point is, that touching people the same way can have different meanings at different times. It is important that you know what you are doing and saying with your touching so that if someone gets the wrong (perhaps sexual) message, you are able to tell them that you have a different intention. Arguments and fights as well as legal action have sometimes started with a misunderstanding about touching.

Your work may require you to touch people, by lifting, feeding, caring for their toilet needs or helping them to walk. This sort of touching is an essential part of the work, as the job would not get done without it. There are, however, different ways of touching people in these circumstances. It is possible to lift gently or roughly, to feed someone in a way that leaves as much of their dignity intact as possible or to do it in a careless sloppy way. It is possible to show understanding in the way you wash someone, but washing them another way could leave them feeling hopeless and dependent.

Scenario

Imagine one of your friends says to you:

> 'I am fed up and angry at my mother. She doesn't seem to understand me, she always complains about the state of my room and my hair, she doesn't like my clothes or my friends; in fact I wonder whether she likes me at all.'

How do you respond? Different methods of response include using minimal prompts, paraphrasing, summarising, and asking open and closed questions.

Minimal prompts

A *probe* is a combination of an open question and a statement which invites further comment. A probe appropriate to the example above could be: 'You said you were angry at your mother'. This is not really a question, but can have the same effect since it invites someone to say more about a specific aspect of what they have told you. The advantage of a probe over a question is that it is easier for someone to ignore if they want to.

A *prompt* is used in most conversation when someone seems a bit stuck. It reminds them that you are there listening to them; e.g. 'Go on', or 'Mmm'. Non-verbal messages which work as prompts can be a nod with the head or a sort of circular motion with the hand.

Prompts need to be used carefully and

sparingly or they will have the opposite effect. Imagine (or remember) what it would be like to have someone nodding away when you need time to explain something complicated. It would make you feel rushed and not listened to.

Later on there will be some practical examples where you will be able to practice these different elements of a helping relationship and identify them as they occur when you observe role-plays.

Paraphrasing

Paraphrasing involves some reflection, but with more input. Not only are you reflecting back, you are also saying something again in a shorter way. Using the example above, a response could be:

> 'It sounds like you feel angry and misunderstood by your mother.'

When you paraphrase, you will often have to leave something out. What you include will depend on what seems important to the person you are helping. You may need to rely on non-verbal clues to get a sense of this.

The girl in the example above might look angry and misunderstood so you would include those feelings in your paraphrasing. If, however, she started to cry when wondering whether her mother likes her at all, you might suggest that she seems to feel sad and rejected.

When paraphrasing, it is more important to include the feelings communicated in a spoken as well as non-verbal way rather than literally what is just said.

Summarising

This involves bringing together what has been said to you and letting the person know that you understand. This can be done by reflective listening and interpreting:

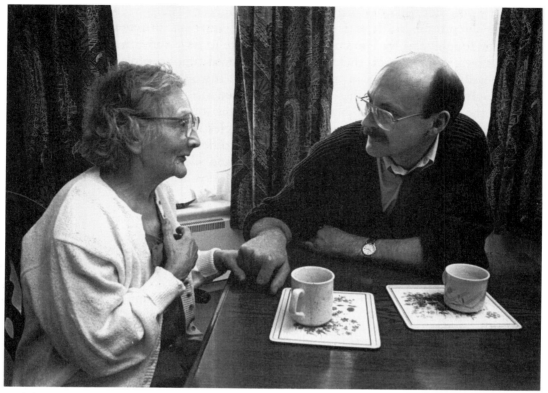

Figure 4.4   *Being a good listener can take time and practice*

REFLECTIVE LISTENING

This involves taking a part of what someone has said and repeating it back to them. There is no right answer here, but in general you are more likely to be perceived as understanding if you reflect back the feeling part of a statement; e.g. 'You sound angry', or 'you feel your mother doesn't seem to understand you'.

Reflecting back may seem like stating the obvious, but it is surprising how you sometimes do not really know what you have said until someone has repeated it back to you.

When reflecting back to a person it is useful to include statements such as: 'It sounds like . . .' or 'I wonder if . . .' or 'Perhaps you . . .' This leaves the person you are helping in control and able to correct or adjust her statement about herself.

INTERPRETING

This involves digging a little deeper and includes making links with what you might know about a person from before. For example: 'It seems that you are angry at your mother and she does not appear to understand you, but I wonder if she feels the same about you?'

You can immediately see that this is quite a big step from reflecting back and paraphrasing because it is based on something which is not in the original statement. Interpretation should therefore be used only very occasionally and certainly not at all until you have spent some time with a person whom you are helping. The problem is that you might be very wrong, which is not so bad if you are trusted, but could undo the early stages of trust if used too soon.

Sometimes you can get a hunch or feeling about someone, and be correct with an interpretation which can be very helpful, but it does involve the risk of being wrong.

Open and closed questions

A closed question usually has only a limited number of answers. For example, 'That's a smart car isn't it?' (closed question) invites a yes or no response; as opposed to 'What do you think of Karen's car?' (open question) which invites you to consider how you feel about the car and comment accordingly.

A closed question is not as useful in a caring relationship because it places a restriction on the person you are trying to care for. Imagine what it must be like to have something important you want to say, but feel embarrassed, hoping you might get the chance to say it, but can't because you keep having to answer questions which have nothing to do with how you are feeling.

Open questions often start with: 'Perhaps you . . . ?' or 'Maybe . . . ?' or 'Possibly you are . . . ?'

When you are asking an open question, you are reflecting back and paraphrasing at the same time, but also hinting that someone might just open up a little more about something.

Of course there are going to be times when you have to ask closed questions, e.g. when you are filling in a form. But generally, you will find that if you keep closed questions to a minimum, you will discover much more about the people you are caring for.

Tone, pitch and pace of communication

Speech is one of the most important parts of a conversation, but it is not just what is said that matters, as sometimes how things are said communicates more. For example almost anything said angrily is more likely to communicate anger rather than what is meant by the words. If you say: 'How are you?' in a warm and friendly way then you convey warmth and friendship. If, on the other hand, you say 'How are you?' in a cool, disinterested way then it is likely that you will communicate the fact that you are not that interested in that person.

DIFFERENT CONTEXTS

Communication skills are used in a number of different settings. So far we have only considered 'one to one'. Communicating in a group is important because we exist in groups. What is a group? There are a number of answers to this but for the purposes of this chapter I will suggest one:

A collection of three or more people with something in common.

What they have in common may be that they are living together in the same house, that they play the same sports together or they share a similar disability. Your fellow students and yourself are a group, although there are likely to be a number of smaller sub-groups of friends within the main group.

Groups are more than just a collection of people; they have an identity of their own. Each member of the group will influence and be influenced by the group. Imagine you are in a group of ten on holiday and a loud majority decide to go to try a local restaurant. You may prefer plain English food but do not want to be the odd one out and end up on your own in a strange town, so you go along with it. If there were just two or three of you it might have been possible to discuss your point of view more easily, but as it is you are outnumbered so you keep your views to yourself.

In this way individual members of a group can be influenced by the majority view, sometimes changing their minds about things they like or believe in.

Another effect of being in a group is that we can experience a sense of belonging, of being a part of something. We can also experience intense rivalry and competitiveness in a group situation. Trying to be heard in a large group is much harder than in a small one, so some members of a group may try to be dominant and attempt to lead the group.

It is important to remember that the dominant members of a group, while appearing very confident, are sometimes quite insecure or worried below the surface. Persuading them to express how they feel beneath the surface will help to prevent them taking over the group.

Some members of the group may feel intimidated or scared to speak out and become very quiet. These individuals may, like the loud ones, be quite worried inside, and will also be helped if they too can express how they feel when they are ready to do so.

Activity 7

 The group is to stand in the middle of a cleared room. The task is now to organise yourself into tall people and short people and see what happens.

COMMENT

 What happened and why? You will probably see how some people describe

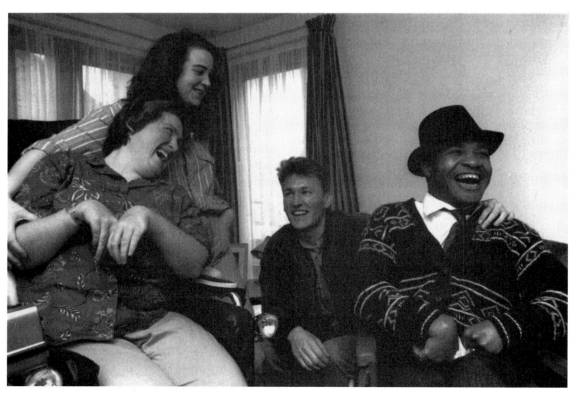

Figure 4.5   *Good communication in a care setting is important for the carer and the client*

themselves as short or tall, and are not challenged. Others who think they are short may be told by members of the group that they are in the wrong group and should be in the tall group. Some people might find that they are not allowed entry to either group as they are not short or tall enough. These people might then form a third 'middle size' group.

Doing this activity will give you an impression of how easily your own views can be challenged and changed by a group. It can seem as if the group has a mind of its own.

OBSERVATION SKILLS

A key to good communication is the ability to *observe*. We learn by watching others as well as ourselves. We observe things all the time, but how much do we think about what we see? There is an important difference between passive and active observation. Passive observation occurs when we see things and do not necessarily think about what we see; e.g. how much do you remember the interaction around you on your last bus or train journey? Probably not as much as you would if you were *actively* observing what was going on around you, thinking about what people really meant, what their concerns were, and whether or not they were communicating those thoughts and feelings to each other.

Activity 8

Get into groups of three and take it in turns to be an observer. The pair to be observed are to take it in turn to tell the other about a recent event where they became angry. (If you are unobtrusive they will probably forget about you after a few minutes.)

Hold a piece of A4 paper horizontally. Draw two lines to divide it into three columns. Record the speaker on your left in the left hand column and the right hand speaker in the right hand column. In the middle space write down all you can about what is happening in their interaction. When something is said, is it a probe or prompt, a paraphrase, an open or closed question? What body language is being used, and why? Is there enough eye contact (without staring)? How does the person telling the story feel, and is she/he being accurately heard by the listener?

The observer is to keep time and allow each person 10 minutes to talk, before stopping them and feeding back their observations. You will probably find that you (as the observer) will have noticed many things which neither the speaker nor listener were aware of. By sharing your observations you will help the couple to develop better communication skills.

COMMENT

By observing communication *actively* you will improve your observation skills by understanding and remembering more of what you see. *Active observation involves thinking about what you see in as many ways as you can.*

OBSTACLES TO EFFECTIVE COMMUNICATION

You may have noticed some obstacles to your efforts to carry out some of the suggested activities so far. We probably communicate best when we can clearly hear and understand each other and when there is a minimum of distractions.

Try Activity 7 above, but instead of being an observer, be a distracter. Wander round the couple talking and fidgeting to yourself. The couple will soon find that communication becomes considerably more difficult.

Environmental obstacles

This includes anything in your immediate surroundings which distracts you from effective communication. Examples are:

- bright lights and direct sunlight
- other people talking
- music being played
- doors and windows left open, letting in the cold
- hard uncomfortable seats

Most of these obstacles can be either removed or minimised, and it is well worth doing this *first* rather than wait until communication becomes difficult.

Bad language and slang

It is sometimes difficult to understand someone when they have a strong accent, speak very quickly, indistinctly or use bad language and slang. You can of course ask someone to slow down, repeat what they have said and speak a bit louder. It is rather more difficult to stop someone using bad language and slang without making them feel either angry or rejected. It is probably best to try to understand as much as you can, possibly asking for clarification now and again. Of course if the bad language is too difficult to bear, you should say so.

If you can understand the feelings behind the words and let the person know you have understood, you will probably find that the need to use bad language disappears.

EVALUATING YOUR OWN COMMUNICATION SKILLS

Activity 9

Take a partner (preferably someone you do not know well). Taking it in turns to be carer and client, tell each other what you do not like about yourself, your body, or your situation. (Before you start it might be a good idea to discuss confidentiality, as you may want to keep what you disclose to each other between yourselves.)

When you are the carer, remember the elements of communication (discussed above) perhaps just starting with reflective listening before moving on to the others. Try not to hurry your partner and remember that he or she will need time to think, so some silences may help, even if they seem a little uncomfortable at first. Remember also to comment on feelings as well as facts even if it seems uncomfortable. By doing this you will be demonstrating that you are open to all his or her communications.

When you are role-playing the person being cared for, remember that you do not have to say anything that you do not want to. Ask yourself how safe you feel; how easy is it to talk about your weak points, the things you are not good at, things you are embarrassed about or feelings of being let down or rejected by someone.

At the end of each turn give your carer some feedback on how it felt, suggesting how they might improve the quality of communication they provide. Remember this is a chance for you to care for each other and not about getting things right or wrong. Questions to ask the person being listened to:

- What needs did you have during this exercise?
- What did you need from your carer?
- How did you feel, sharing something about yourself which you did not like?

The following are some answers I thought of:
- Being accepted as you are.
- Not being judged.
- Being understood.
- Being given the space and time to collect together thoughts and feelings.
- Someone to trust.

Questions to ask the carer:
- Could you accept this person as they were and not try to give advice or feel disapproving?
- Could you be open to all their communications without trying to alter what they were trying to say to you?

SUMMARY

Everybody has particular needs, depending on their circumstances. An elderly person who is in a residential home and mourning her husband needs someone to understand how much she misses him and how lonely and sad she feels. Another example is a young man who has been paralysed below the waist. He might feel angry at the world for robbing him of an active life, embarrassed and helpless at having to depend on someone to help him go to the lavatory.

Both these people need to feel better about themselves; they need to be cared for by a person who understands the importance of good communication. It is of very little value trying to convince such a person that things will brighten up. Doing this is often a way of avoiding difficult and painful feelings in someone else. Think of the way we greet each other. 'Hi, how are you?' is usually met by something like: 'Fine thanks'.

It is much more difficult to say: 'Well, since you ask, I've got a headache, I'm behind with my work and I'm fed up with my Mum.' You may get the response: 'Oh well, if that is how you feel, it's not going to be much fun around here, so I'll go and find someone more cheerful.' Of course you may be lucky and have a friend who puts her needs for a cheerful friend to one side, so she can try to understand your needs.

Although the communication skills you will need differ from person to person, the ways in which we can be helpful do not vary much. Look back to the communication skills which were useful in the Activity 9 above.

If 'the carer' was being skilful she would probably have been:

- observant, looking out for non-verbal messages which give a clue as to how you feel about what you are saying.
- non-judgemental, so you could be open about how you feel even if some of the feelings are negative, like anger or sadness.
- able to accept you as an individual, however different you may be from your carer.
- using the conversational elements (or parts) of the caring relationship appropriately (such as reflective listening, open questions and paraphrasing).

The important point to remember is that skilful communication is not necessarily a normal part of conversation. It is quite easy to be lonely in a crowd or at a party. Good communication requires an effort. It involves thinking for another person and does not always come naturally. It takes time and practice to get used to, so do not expect to be able to do it right away, although by now you should be on the right track.

Interpersonal relationships and discrimination

INTRODUCTION

Discrimination involves policies and practices which exclude people from certain groups on the basis of, for example, their gender, age, disabilities or ethnic origin. These policies may be explicit, where a job advertisement excludes certain groups, for example by saying that only those aged between 25 and 35 need apply. They may be less explicit where there is no published age limit, but only those of a certain age are shortlisted.

Groups of people such as women, people aged between 40 and 50, black people and disabled people, talk about there being a 'glass ceiling', which prevents them from career progression. It is important that people are selected for work on the basis of their ability to do the job. In order to prevent discrimination when working with or caring for people from different ethnic backgrounds it is important to ensure that their specific needs are met, such as the kinds of food they do or do not eat. Spiritual beliefs, customs and values should be respected and efforts should be made to ensure that everyone is aware of different needs.

Abuse is another manifestation of prejudice and includes various forms such as verbal and physical abuse. Abuse seriously restricts people from being able to lead their 'normal' lifestyle. It is necessary to respect people as individuals and to speak up for them if they are not able to do so for themselves, in order to prevent hurtful attitudes and violence. Sometimes violence and abuse are taken to extremes. When countries are at war, people are often killed because of their ethnic origin. Abuse continues to occur in troubled areas throughout the world. Amnesty International is one organisation which attempts to draw attention to it.

DIFFERENT FORMS OF DISCRIMINATION

There are many ways in which we discriminate against others. The basis of discrimination is *difference*. We cannot help noticing the difference between ourselves and other people. There is no harm in simply noticing a difference. People come in all sorts of different sizes, shapes, ages, colours, abilities, sexual preferences and so on. The problems start when we think that one such size, colour or ability is *better* than the other. This is negative discrimination. In order to make ourselves feel more secure in our identity, we discriminate between ourselves and others so that we are superior in some way. Although this makes us *feel* superior it has the unfortunate effect of making the other person feel as though they are *made* to be inferior, when they are not. They will therefore feel angry, upset and humiliated.

Imagine how someone who is bullied at school feels; you will get some idea of the effect of negative discrimination.

Discrimination affects interpersonal relationships in a number of ways. We cannot avoid getting older, yet increasingly in our culture old age is represented as boring, shabby, not well, 'wrinkly', 'out of it', and a bit 'sad'. By contrast youth is represented as 'in', vibrant, strong, energetic, sexy and the best way to be. Now while some of this may well be true, these labels have become a stereotype. Can you think of some boring young people and some energetic old people? We have come to regard old age as something that we must accept, rather than a time of wisdom and reflection. Ageism is a common feature of the workplace, with people being sacked because they are considered too old to carry out their jobs, even when they can demonstrate that the accumulated experience of the years actually makes them better than their younger competitors.

We all differ in our abilities and state of health. Some are stronger, less agile, clever, artistic, unmusical, can't walk, can't see, etc. Some less able people have a restricted access to parts of life which most people would regard as a basic right, such as using the bus, going to the cinema, or using the lavatory. Many people with a disability would point out that it is bad enough having a disability without being deprived of parts of life to which the more able have access. One way disabled persons can obtain greater access to areas they are kept out of, is through effective communication. This may be difficult for them, and their carers need to *adapt their communication skills* to the needs of the disabled and unwell so their efforts to communicate are effective.

get access to middle and higher management jobs than it is for men. The same applies to ethnic and racial minorities. There are public misconceptions of links between crime and race, as there are misconceptions about links between gender and leadership qualities. Personal beliefs, such as religion or politics, can be the basis for negative discrimination. Some religions require certain customs to be followed, such as the wearing of special clothes, or headwear. Others, not fully understanding the religious meaning of these forms of dress, may treat such persons with suspicion or hostility. Sometimes differences like this can get in the way of effective interpersonal relationships without us being able to help it. What does help is to think about our attitudes to difference so that we are aware of how relationships can be affected by discriminatory behaviour.

The next activity calls on you to consider your attitudes in relation to sexuality. For some people this can be uncomfortable or embarrassing. One way of dealing with this difficulty is to trivialise the topic and 'laugh it off'. This is a way of saying 'I can't handle this and therefore it is a waste of time'. As a carer you may be faced with a scenario like the following one, and you will be much better able to care for the person if you have worked through some of your own discomfort. This will make all the difference for the person you are caring for.

Activity 10

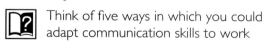 Think of five ways in which you could adapt communication skills to work effectively with someone who is disabled or unwell.

We cannot do much to change our race or gender, yet we can be treated very differently as a result of these differences. For example, it is still much more difficult for women to

Activity 11

 This activity can be used as an assignment or discussed in your group.

Imagine you are working in a residential home for children aged between 10 and 16. One of the girls approaches you and tells you she is attracted to other girls.

Ask yourselves the following questions and think about your answers in terms of prejudices you may have.

- How does this make you feel?
- Are you able to accept her as she is?
- What do you think she needs from you?
- How do you think she is feeling?

COMMENT

 Remember, we all have prejudices, sometimes without knowing it. It can be difficult to accept our prejudices; usually they are a way of avoiding the things about ourselves which we do not like.

BEHAVIOURS WHICH MAY INDICATE DISCRIMINATION

We can usually see when someone is discriminating against a person. Someone who is being deprived of a right or service they are entitled to for reasons of their difference, is a victim of discrimination. It is possible that all sorts of justification will be given to support such an action, rather than give the genuine reason (prejudice). By law, there are basically two types of discrimination: direct and indirect. Direct discrimination is a rule or attitude which explicitly excludes one group, e.g. 'only men may apply', or 'under 25s only'. This is usually quite easy to spot. Indirect discrimination occurs when a rule that applies equally to everybody has the effect of discriminating against one group. Sometimes rules which appear fair can be misinterpreted by someone who is discriminating against an individual or group, as the following scenario indicates.

Scenario

You are in a residential home where vegetarian requests are normally catered for. You overhear a care worker arguing with a resident. She (the care worker) is red in the face

and getting quite angry. The resident is an elderly Japanese man who looks close to tears. Listening a while longer you learn that one of the residents, Mr Chung, has asked not to have the minced beef on offer for supper. Katie, the care worker is getting worked up because Mr Chung has eaten meat before and therefore is not considered a vegetarian. She does not agree with his reasons for asking for fish on this occasion and sees him as a silly old foreigner. Mr Chung sees Katie as someone who refuses to understand his culture as different to her own and feels rejected and quite upset.

Activity 12

Try role-playing the scenario in front of your group.
After the role-play ask yourselves the following questions:
- How is Katie discriminating against Mr Chung?
- What behaviour indicates her discrimination?
- What can Katie do to improve the relationship between herself and Mr Chung?

COMMENT

Katie is discriminating against Mr Chung by not giving him the same rights and service as the other residents. She is discriminating against him *indirectly* by implying that he 'ought' to be like the others. Her angry attitude gives away her real prejudices against people who are different. She is suggesting that she can accept vegetarians but not others with specific food preferences.

There are a number of ways we reveal indirect discrimination. Imagine you are in a conversation in a group and the topic moves to homosexuality. Someone mentions the dilemma of a gay friend who is considering coming out and you find yourself changing the subject to a holiday you recently had with a boyfriend (or a girlfriend if you are male). What does this change of subject suggest to you? We often reveal our true feelings to ourselves; we are sometimes the first or only ones to spot these behaviours which indicate prejudice and discrimination in ourselves, and can *learn from the experience*. If you spot this type of indirect discrimination in someone else it is probably more effective to try to open up the discussion than confront them directly. If they feel they are in the wrong they are likely to become defensive and attempt to justify their prejudices.

STEREOTYPING AND DISCRIMINATORY BEHAVIOUR

Individuality: We are all different!

We are all different in many ways, and the differences we see between ourselves and others may not be the same differences that others see between themselves and us. We live in a world where differences are more noticeable as people from various races, upbringing, culture and belief are coming together and living in communities. Travel and trading links have made the world seem a smaller place than at any time in our history. The differences between people are frequently given as the cause for tension and conflict;

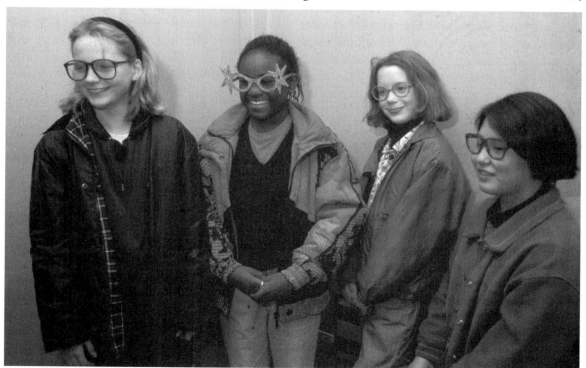

Figure 4.6   *Race is not a barrier to friendship*

you need only think of the many wars taking place to see this.

What differences between people can you think of? Before going any further make a list of as many differences that you can think of.

Some of these might include: age, sex, race, colour, height, weight, physical ability, mental ability, religion, favourite football team, hair colour, attitudes, sexuality.

Consider what you like about your friends for a moment. An important factor is probably sharing something in common. This could include things you like to do, e.g. sports, going out together, the area you live in, a sense of humour, smoking, dancing and many more. When you are friends you may not notice some of the differences listed above. If you do, I would imagine that you can make a joke about some of them. Although only 'jokes', these differences can sometimes hurt when people draw attention to them, even when they are friends. People who are unfriendly frequently use differences as a way of making others feel uncomfortable, frightened or hurt.

It is as though people who are being unfriendly or hostile are trying to make other people feel bad so they can feel good about themselves (when in fact they might feel quite bad about themselves).

All the 'isms' such as racism, sexism, or ageism are a part of this process, which contributes to prejudice. Those who attack others (either physically or verbally) because of their differences, usually do not feel very good about themselves, and have low self-esteem. Since all of us can occasionally feel bad about ourselves, we are all open to some sort of prejudice.

Have you noticed how someone who expresses some sort of prejudice, such as a racist joke, or making fun of someone who is disabled or old, is usually trying to win you round to their point of view, so they can feel good about themselves at the expense of their 'victims'? Although a part of you might feel it is cruel to enjoy the suffering of others, it can be difficult to resist, especially if you are a minority of one in a group all laughing at someone's expense. The reason it is difficult to resist is that we end up being the odd one out, so it is sometimes easier to go along with the majority than take a risk of being different.

Understanding individuality is very important in helping relationships since you may be working with people of all ages, religions, races and abilities. The ability to provide emotional support will depend on the extent to which you consider those you are helping as individual people and not as just 'old', 'disabled' or 'black'. Some of the people you work with may feel the odd one out; part of the job of meeting their care needs (helping them to feel better about themselves) is to understand how they feel and accept them as they are. Whether you are working in a hospital or in a care situation, you will be with people who are to some extent dependant on assistance from others.

Some people may seem very different on the outside, but when you get in touch with how they feel it is surprising how similar we all are. The feelings of pain, rejection, sadness and happiness are all there below the surface, provided you listen for them.

Stereotyping groups

So far we have looked at discriminatory behaviour in terms of individuals, so let us now look at the effect of thinking about groups as stereotypes. Stereotyping is what we do when we 'label' an individual or group without seeing what they are really like. Can you think of any examples of stereotyping groups?

Examples are:

'Groups of young white men with very short hair, tattoos and high boots are skinheads and therefore likely to attack Asians.'

While this may be true in some cases it is clearly unfair to the many people for whom it is not true.

'Women are weaker than men and therefore should not work on building sites.'

Again this is clearly not necessarily true. The statement hides all sorts of assumptions our culture has about femininity and the way men maintain control of the workplace. This is particularly true of an area which men try to keep as exclusively 'macho'.

Groups have a life of their own, and need to find something similar about all the members. This becomes part of their identity and is important to the group. From the outside the 'badges' of identity (tattoos, spiky hair, body piercing as well as particular attitudes) can seem to exclude us. Feeling left out, we tend to strike back and make generalisations about other people on the basis of their appearance or attitudes in an attempt to feel less left out and more secure.

COMMENT

ⓘ We need to make generalisations to survive and make sense of the world around us. Unfortunately we tend to make generalisations about people in the way we group them together. How often have you heard something like: 'Well everybody knows that all ... are ... !' If we do this as carers, we fail to see people as individuals and run the risk of providing a low standard of care.

POSSIBLE EFFECTS OF DISCRIMINATION

If you agree with what has been said so far about discrimination, then it is likely that you will try to reduce discriminatory behaviour by yourself and those around you. Unfortunately we are not always in the position of being able to do something about it ourselves and may be working with an individual who has suffered the effects of discrimination by others. What are these effects and what can we do to help?

Short-term effects

When someone is discriminated against, they are effectively deprived of something which they could reasonably expect as a right. When something is taken away from you what is your first reaction? Probably anger. This anger may be on the surface as angry behaviour, finding fault with anything and everything, or it may lurk below the surface as stress, causing illness and depression.

Long-term effects

Over a period of time discrimination may lead to a belief that if a person is not getting something that they are entitled to, it must be because they are worthless (low sense of self-worth, a feeling of worthlessness). These feelings can lead such a person to depression and stress-induced illness. If a person believes they have less worth they may be less effective in getting work.

EQUAL OPPORTUNITY RIGHTS

There are a number of laws which deal with 'equal opportunity rights'. They exist so that a person can receive support if they become a victim of discrimination, and are intended to deter employers and others from behaving in a discriminatory fashion. In general there are a number of Acts of Parliament which refer to sex discrimination, equal pay, race relations, and disability. These Acts are designed to protect the rights of individuals in a number of key areas including:

- employment and training
- education
- the provision of goods and services
- pay
- financial services
- tenancy
- access to leisure facilities

There are penalties for those who break these laws as well as rights of appeal for those who, for example, are barred from certain jobs on

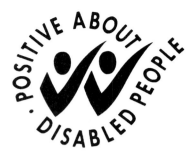

Figure 4.7   *This logo shows that employers offer equal opportunities for disabled people*

the basis of race, gender or age. If successful on appeal, an employer may have to accept someone back into the workforce, or in other cases pay them the same amount as others doing the same job. There are still a number of areas where there is no legislation against discrimination, such as the prison service, some areas of policing, and immigration control.

Aspects of working with clients

THE CARING RELATIONSHIP

The caring relationship differs from other relationships in a number of ways. There are voluntary and paid caring relationships. A daughter caring for an elderly and housebound parent has a different type of caring relationship from a paid care worker in a residential home. Although there is much in common in practice between the two types of relationship, it is important to remember that when we are being paid for something, we are in effect agreeing to carry out certain tasks and services to a required standard. This means that there is the element of a *contract* in a caring relationship. It is a professional relationship which has certain clear boundaries and although it may be friendly

it is primarily a working relationship and not a friendship. The caring relationship has a *purpose*. This will involve guaranteeing that the client will get the service they are entitled to: part of that service is a high standard of interpersonal relationship which recognises the client's needs and puts them first. To do this effectively it helps to develop communication skills, but this is not enough on its own. An awareness of client rights and ethical issues (see below), a knowledge of the effects of discrimination and a willingness to recognise and support the needs of the client are also very important.

Scenario

Joy

You work in a residential home for young children up to nine years old. One of the staff, Joy, has asked to have a quiet talk with you; she seems worried so you agree and find a small room to meet in after lunch. Joy tells you that one of the children's parents has made a formal complaint about her. The manager of the home has said that the complaint is being investigated and will probably lead to a disciplinary tribunal fixed to take place in four weeks time. In the meantime Joy has been moved to another part of the home where she will have no contact with the little boy concerned (who is seven). Joy tells you, through angry tears, that she is alleged to have hit the boy hard with a spoon during a meal. Joy tells you that she tapped him lightly with the spoon on the back of his hand because he had grabbed some food from another child's plate and started throwing it all over the other children. She complains that this boy has been terribly disruptive recently and that efforts to move him to another special unit have failed due to budget restrictions at the end of the financial year.

Joy is angry with the parent who believes the word of a disruptive child without consulting her to find out what really happened. She is angry with the management for allowing the situation to get out of hand by not dealing with the situation in the first place, and now for seeming to take sides against her. She is frightened about losing her job, which would be disastrous since she is a single parent and receives no maintenance from her little girl's father.

- How would you care for Joy?
- How does her story make you feel?
- Are you able to help her by understanding how she feels without giving her advice or 'taking sides'? In other words, can you help her reach her own solution?

HOW CLIENTS MAY RESPOND TO RECEIVING CARE

The way clients respond to our care provision will give us a good idea as to the quality of care we are providing. Assuming (and this is not always the case) that the agreed service is adequate for the needs of your client group, then your clients are likely to respond in a positive way to your care: they will be pleased, impressed perhaps, maybe grateful and you will be rewarded with positive feedback. Of course this is not always the case, and there will be some clients who will be unhappy and angry however hard you try. It is easy to be put off by such behaviour and tempting to be angry back which will usually make matters worse. Try understanding where the anger or upset comes from without 'labelling' the client. In addition to this you could talk to other staff about your feelings; being understood yourself will make it easier to understand your clients.

Scenario 2

The rehabilitation centre

You work in a rehabilitation centre for people recovering from major illness or accident. Some of the residents have been there for a long time, and although the centre runs smoothly for most of the time, there is a growing feeling of resentment among the long stay residents at some of the changes that have been taking place recently. The number of staff has been reduced in a cost-cutting exercise, which has made it difficult to give the attention that was given before. The kitchen staff who were previously employed by the health authority have been sacked and some of them re-employed by a catering firm to save money. One result of this is that the food is more boring than it used to be, consisting mainly of chips and pre-packaged food which is re-heated. As there are fewer kitchen staff than before, the meals are staggered over a longer period, meaning that it is difficult for residents to get their meals at the same time each day.

Seven of the residents have formed an action group to change things and your manager has asked you to meet them to hear their grievances. They will be hoping that you can change things, but you know that the budget cuts means that the situation is more likely to worsen than improve.

Feeling quite nervous you start the meeting by saying that you cannot make any promises, but hope to be able to discuss the issues and try to improve the situation within existing resources.

Members of the group angrily say that they feel let down and ignored, and direct much of their frustration at you.

- What are the care needs of the group?
- How can you care for them without giving in to their demands?
- What communication skills enable you to do this?
- Can you avoid 'taking sides' and becoming angry with the group or with the management (even if part of you wants to)?

Scenario 3

In the same residential home as Scenario 2, imagine that you are called in to help resolve a dispute that has developed about which TV channel to watch. One group wants to watch Brookside, but a smaller group wants to watch a wildlife programme on a different side. There is only one TV and no video.

- Does it help to tell the children which programme you think they ought to watch?
- What can you do to help the group reach

some sort of decision without a riot?
- How do you avoid seeming to take sides?

SUPPORT AND THE CLIENT/CARER RELATIONSHIP

Every person has a right to benefit from the services which are appropriate to their needs. This means that they must know about different services available to them, and understand how to apply for the service. They must be able to contact the relevant person or obtain the appropriate application form. To ensure the maximum accessibility of this service, everyone should be provided with access to a telephone or transport, and information leaflets in a language they can understand. Finally, everyone has a right not to be discriminated against in receiving health or care services on account of race, sex, age, disability or any reason. See Chapter 3, pages 96–97 for further discussion of this issue.

CONFIDENTIALITY AND ETHICAL ISSUES

A professional person providing social care, e.g. a social worker or a care assistant, gets to know a lot of very personal information about their client, and may be involved in giving some quite intimate personal care. It is essential that the information is kept confidential and not talked about without the client's permission.

Some information may need to be passed from one professional to another, from one care worker to another or to a nurse, social worker or doctor, but this must be done with the client's permission.

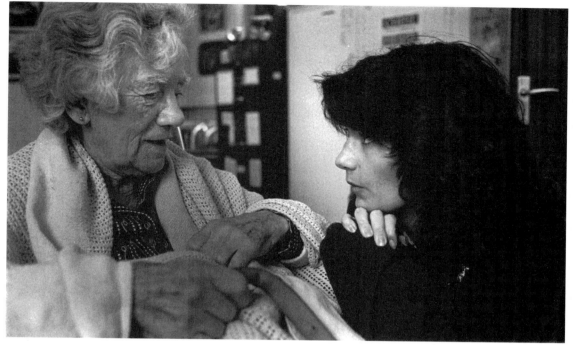

Figure 4.8   *It is essential for a client to be able to trust the carer*

There are usually clear guidelines for the exchange of this type of information, and rights for the client to have access to any records that are kept on them. Part of your job may include ensuring your client is granted these rights of privacy and access.

Close relationships may develop between clients and their care workers, and even when conversations are informal, it is important to regard them as confidential. These relationships should be friendly and informal but still remain professional.

There are times when difficulties can arise.

Activity 13

Suppose you are talking with a neighbour one evening and learn that one of her friends is a young disabled woman who you care for. You learn that your client is being abused by a step-father but does not want to discuss it or report it. She fears this may make things worse. You are aware that your client has been tearful and upset lately and you were wondering why. Your neighbour has told you this in confidence and does not know of your professional relationship with the disabled girl.

How can you help the girl without breaking confidentiality or going against the wishes of your client? Discuss this in small groups of three and try to arrive at some suggestions. Take turns to present your suggestions to the larger group. Do not be surprised to find a wide difference of opinion.

COMMENT

Please remember that there are no right answers to this. It is a difficult situation which should be thought through very carefully before action (if any) is taken. Some work settings provide confidential professional supervision which should be sought if this is available. It should be possible to discuss your dilemma here without breaking confidences (you can discuss clients without revealing names). The important thing is to not act impulsively on your own as this will almost certainly worsen things, however bad they may be. Seeking professional help and support in difficult situations is the responsible and wise thing to do.

Summary

We have looked at how interpersonal relationships can be affected by discrimination. Discrimination is all about not tolerating difference, and seems to occur everywhere to some extent. The effects of discrimination can be very damaging and we therefore need to think about it in order to be aware of it when and where it occurs. It is easy to come to the conclusion that it is only other people who discriminate. Somehow we do easily not notice the way we cannot help discriminating by being part of systems and institutions which offer rights, services and goods in an unequal way (depending on age, sex, race, ability etc.).

There are different types of discrimination: we have looked at direct discrimination which is easier to spot, as well as indirect discrimination which can go unnoticed by many. When we are faced with difference we sometimes stereotype others; in so doing, we fail to see them as individuals and our relationship with them will suffer accordingly. While this applies to any relationship, it is especially true for a caring relationship.

The final topic was confidentiality. Maintaining confidentiality can sometimes be a burden on a care worker so please remember to consult a senior when you are not sure what is expected of you.

DEFINITIONS

The following is a list of definitions of some of the 'jargon' terms used in the performance criteria. They are taken from the performance criteria as they occur and while you are not expected to learn them at this stage, (further explanations will follow) it would be helpful to read them through now while referring to the performance criteria so you know where to look if you want to define a particular term.

Body language Non-verbal language, communicating with posture gestures, facial expressions, eye contact and sometimes touching.

Caring relationship Any relationship where one person has the task of helping another, such as a caring or nursing role. Recognising and understanding a person's feelings (such as anger, fear, sadness, confusion, gratitude, envy, love and guilt), followed by an effort to understand their needs (such as love, understanding, honesty, practical help, comfort, food, warmth, respect and care). This includes actually meeting someone's needs and/or helping them to express their needs in a way which can be understood by others.

Closed question A question which limits the number of possible answers: e.g. 'Are you upset?' is a closed question which can be answered with a yes or no.

Confidentiality Keeping things private. In a professional sense it means respecting the *rights* to confidentiality that clients have. Confidentiality has certain limitations, especially in cases where crimes are thought to be occurring. Employers should give clear guidelines about any limitations.

Conversational techniques Specially adapted ways in which we communicate to another person, in order to help them. This involves putting the other person's needs above our own. Not just a conversation where you both talk about yourselves, but the use of conversation (talking and listening) to understand and help. Conversational techniques form part of the helping relationship.

Discrimination   In practice this means *negative* discrimination when a person deprives another of a right on the basis of race, age, sex, religion, disability or any other difference.

Empathy   The ability to understand another person's feelings from their own point of view by using your own feelings to enter their world imaginatively. Not to be confused with sympathy, where you sometimes guess you know how someone feels because you think you have had the same experience yourself.

Ethics   Codes or professional practice, how to behave according to established rules within a profession or by law.

Evidence indicators   What the students need to show to demonstrate their understanding of the unit. This could include written or practical presentations (for example discussions and role-plays).

Individuality   The extent to which a person is separate and unique. This includes physical characteristics as well as personality. Physical characteristics include appearance, race, age, sex, health, and physical ability/disability. Non-physical characteristics include culture, religion, social group, sexuality, language and mental ability/disability. All these and other factors combine to produce a person's individuality.

Interpreting   A comment which is aimed at trying to understand what someone really means. Interpreting is a skill which can be used when you have got to know someone you are trying to help, who may find it difficult to ask for what they need. For example, being bad tempered may be a way of asking for help. Interpreting is like

translating something into an idea you can both understand.

Non-verbal message   Any form of communication that is not actually spoken. Certain expressions have meanings which we all know about without having to say what is meant: e.g. smiling, frowning, looking tense, looking relaxed, talking gently, talking aggressively.

Open question   A question which enables a person to choose an answer in their own way: e.g. 'I wonder if you are upset?' is an open question which invites a person to consider how they feel. It also communicates to someone a willingness to be flexible.

Paraphrasing   Saying something in another, usually shorter, way. Paraphrasing is often used to summarise something a person has said. This shows that you have heard and understood what has been said and gives the person a chance to think over what they said. Sometimes we are surprised when something we have said is repeated back to us or played back through a recorder.

Performance criteria   An agreed set of standards used to judge the ability to understand and perform a particular task.

Probe   A statement which invites a person to reflect more deeply on what she/he is feeling or saying.

Prompt   A verbal or non verbal way of asking someone to carry on or start communication. A nod, a gesture with the hands or a murmur are examples.

Questioning technique   Any particular way of asking a question.

Range   The limits over which the performance criteria apply.

Reflective listening   Carefully listening to a person and communicating to them that you have heard and understood what she or he has said, without adding your own views or opinions to the reply.

Self-esteem Respect for oneself. Liking oneself 'warts and all'. Self-esteem can be expressed in a feeling of being happy with yourself, even though there may be room for improvement. Low self-esteem often results from a feeling of not being loved for what one is, but loved on condition of being 'good' or 'clever'.

Social interaction The process of two or more people meeting and communicating. This will include conversation as well as non-verbal communication.

Stereotype A fixed view of a person or group on the basis of common characteristics. Views such as 'All French eat frogs' are clearly untrue and based on a stereotype. There are all sorts of stereotypes about minority and disadvantaged groups in British society, which carers will come across.

5

APPLICATION OF SCIENCE IN HEALTH AND SOCIAL CARE

AIMS AND OBJECTIVES

In this chapter, we are going to look at the human body and how it works. If we know how the body normally works, then by making measurements and observations we can detect possible diseases. Even in this technological age, observations can tell us a lot about the physical and mental health of a person.

After completion of this chapter you should understand:

- how the body systems are organised, the functions of those systems, and the relationships between them.

- the measurements and observations that can be made in a care setting to determine the physical and mental health of an individual.

- how scientific principles can be applied in a care setting to increase the comfort of an individual, and aid a carer in the performance of his/her duties.

Cells, tissues, organs and organ systems

All living things are made up of *cells*. Some organisms, for example bacteria, consist of only one cell. Others are made up of many millions of different cells which all work together for the good of the organism.

Cells can differ in size, shape, and function. Specialised cells group together to perform a particular task, and are called *tissues*: e.g.

- nerve tissue is made up of cells capable of carrying nerve impulses

- muscle tissue is composed of cells that will contract and relax

Several different tissues can group to form an *organ*: e.g.

- the heart is made up of muscle, nerves, blood vessels etc.

Organ systems consist of several organs working together: e.g.

- the circulatory system is composed of the heart, blood vessels and blood.

THE BASIC STRUCTURE OF AN ANIMAL CELL

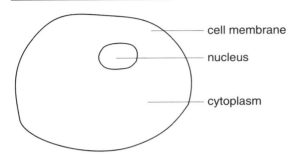

Figure 5.1   *The basic structure of an animal cell*

1 *cell membrane* – controls the entry and exit of substances into and out of the cell

2 *nucleus* – contains the genetic information passed on from the previous generation and regulates the chemical activity of the cell

3 *cytoplasm* – jelly-like fluid containing specialised areas. All the chemical reactions the cell needs to perform to release energy and grow, take place here.

For a cell to obtain energy it needs *oxygen* and food in the form of glucose to be brought to the cell, and these must cross the cell membrane into the cell. Then the following chemical reaction takes place:

$$glucose + oxygen \rightarrow carbon\ dioxide + water + energy$$

The energy can be in the form of heat, or mechanical energy for muscle cell contraction etc.

How does oxygen and glucose get to the cell?

You know we breathe in oxygen and obtain glucose from food, but we should look at these processes in more detail. First, however, we need to look at the different zones the body is divided into.

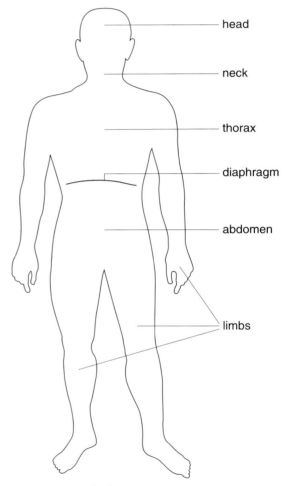

Figure 5.2   *Body zones*

RESPIRATORY SYSTEM

This consists of all the passageways in the

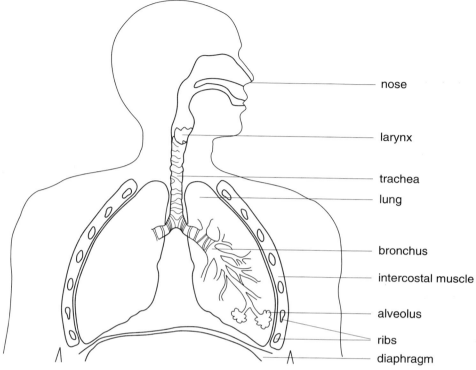

Figure 5.3   *Organs of the respiratory system*

nose, the trachea (the windpipe), the lungs, the ribs and diaphragm.

- *nose* system of passages lined with cells that can produce mucus, and others that have hairs. Together these have a cleansing function.
- *trachea* it is supported by circular bands of tough cartilage to prevent the tube collapsing.
- *lungs* spongy organs which oxygenate the blood and remove carbon dioxide
- *bronchus* branches forming thinner and thinner tubes until they end at the alveoli.
- *alveoli* structure like a bunch of grapes where exchange of gases takes place. The walls are only one cell thick.
- *intercostal muscles* between the ribs.
- *ribs* these form a protective cage around the lungs.

- *diaphragm* a sheet of muscle lining the base of the thorax.

Contraction of the intercostal muscles and the diaphragm expands the chest and inflates the lungs by drawing air into them. Oxygen moves across the cell membrane of the alveoli and into the bloodstream. Carbon dioxide crosses in the opposite direction and is expelled when the muscles relax and breathing out occurs.

The process by which molecules move from where there is a high concentration to where the concentration is low, is called *diffusion*. Both oxygen and carbon dioxide diffuse in the lungs, but in opposite directions.

Oxygen and carbon dioxide are carried around the body to the individual body cells in the bloodstream.

Activity 1

1 Why do you think the alveoli are grape-like structures and not just like a balloon?
2 What do you think will happen to the amount of oxygen in the bloodstream if a person has a breathing disorder or a disease e.g. bronchitis?

(See pages 174–5 for answers to activity questions in this chapter.)

THE CIRCULATORY SYSTEM

This consists of the heart, blood vessels and blood.

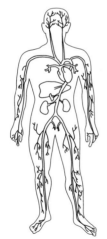

Figure 5.4   *The circulatory system*

It functions as a transport system for:

1 food particles dissolved in the fluid part of the blood (plasma, see page 150)

2 oxygen carried by a special chemical called haemoglobin

3 waste products of metabolism carried from the cell to the kidneys (see page 151)

4 carbon dioxide dissolved in the plasma

5 chemical messengers (hormones) carried from the endocrine gland that produced them to their target organ (see page 156)

6 white cells which have a role in fighting microbes that invade the body

The heart

The heart has four chambers separated down the middle by the septum. The top two chambers are called atria (plural: atrium), and the bottom two, ventricles. Valves between the atria and ventricles, and at the exits to the ventricles prevent back-flow of blood (see Fig. 5.5).

When the heart contracts, the atria contracts first, pushing blood into the ventricles. The ventricles then contract and push blood out of the heart. These two contractions are a fraction of a second apart, and give the characteristic 'lub-dub' sound. Because of its structure, the heart acts as a double pump, with two circulatory pathways, as shown in Fig. 5.6:

• Circulation around the lungs is called the *Pulmonary* Circulation.
• Circulation around the body is called the *Systemic* Circulation.

Arteries

Arteries carry blood away from the heart. Because of the pressure and quantity of blood pulsing through them caused by the pumping action of the heart, arteries need walls containing muscle, so they can expand and contract. As can be seen from Fig. 5.4, the arteries branch out and become smaller and smaller. Eventually they form tubes small enough to pass between the individual cells of the body, and have thin walls so that food and oxygen can pass through them, and

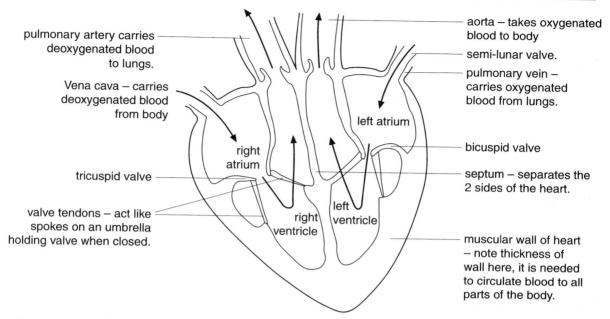

pulmonary artery carries deoxygenated blood to lungs.

Vena cava – carries deoxygenated blood from body

tricuspid valve

valve tendons – act like spokes on an umbrella holding valve when closed.

right atrium

left atrium

right ventricle

left ventricle

aorta – takes oxygenated blood to body

semi-lunar valve.

pulmonary vein – carries oxygenated blood from lungs.

bicuspid valve

septum – separates the 2 sides of the heart.

muscular wall of heart – note thickness of wall here, it is needed to circulate blood to all parts of the body.

Figure 5.5   *The heart*

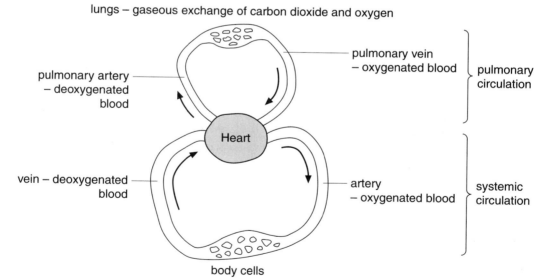

lungs – gaseous exchange of carbon dioxide and oxygen

pulmonary artery – deoxygenated blood

pulmonary vein – oxygenated blood

pulmonary circulation

Heart

vein – deoxygenated blood

artery – oxygenated blood

systemic circulation

body cells

Figure 5.6   *The heart's double circulation*

into the cells. These vessels are called *capillaries*.

Veins

Veins carry blood to the heart. Because the blood has lost the pressure created by the pumping action of the heart, the veins need valves to prevent back-flow of blood. Minute contractions of muscles that surround the veins help blood to be passed along them.

Activity 2

3 Why do the ventricles have thicker walls than the atria?

4 What is the purpose of a valve?

THE DIGESTIVE SYSTEM

This consists of a tube called the *alimentary canal*. This tube is divided into different sections, in order to break down food into very small soluble particles that can be absorbed into the blood stream for transporting to the cells of the body.

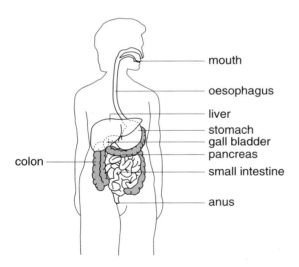

Figure 5.7   *The digestive system*

- *mouth*   physically breaks down food by the chewing action of the teeth. The chemical breakdown of carbohydrates is started by an enzyme called amylase in saliva.

- *oesophagus*   food pipe leading to the stomach
- *stomach*   produces acid which gives the correct conditions for the start of protein digestion by an enzyme called pepsin.
- *pancreas*   produces enzymes that continue carbohydrate and protein breakdown, and lipase (an enzyme to start fat digestion)
- *liver*   produces bile which is stored in the gall bladder
- *gall bladder*   stores bile which emulsifies fats (i.e. works like a detergent, allowing fat and water to mix) and neutralises the acid from the stomach
- *small intestine*   its walls produce enzymes that complete the digestion process. Absorption into the bloodstream of the now soluble food particles also takes place in the lower part
- *colon*   absorbs water and compacts contents
- *rectum*   stores waste ready for elimination
- *anus*   ejects food that cannot be digested from the body

The walls of the intestine are muscular, and waves of contraction called peristalsis move food along. Indigestible parts of plant cell walls (sometimes called dietary fibre) provide bulk and help this process. Too little fibre means that food passes too slowly and constipation results.

- Carbohydrate foods are broken down to simple sugars e.g. glucose.
- Proteins are broken down to amino acids.
- Fats are broken down to fatty acids and glycerol.

All these products of digestion are small, soluble and can be absorbed into the blood stream through the walls of the small intestine.

Villi are small projections of tissue in the small intestine. They increase the surface area

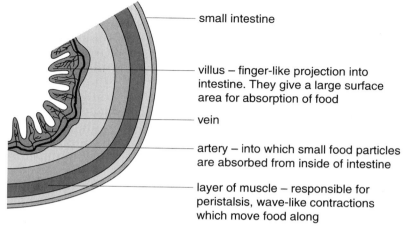

small intestine

villus – finger-like projection into intestine. They give a large surface area for absorption of food

vein

artery – into which small food particles are absorbed from inside of intestine

layer of muscle – responsible for peristalsis, wave-like contractions which move food along

Figure 5.8   *A cross-section through the intestine wall*

available for absorption of digested food.

The last step in digestion is **assimilation** or intake of the digested food into the cells of the body from the blood stream. The food is used to produce energy (carbohydrates and fats), and for growth and repair of the body (proteins). This is called **metabolism.**

When the body uses proteins, it produces waste containing nitrogen. If this was allowed to accumulate in the body, it would poison it, or slow down the rate of metabolism. This waste is removed by the kidneys during excretion.

Diet

To maintain a healthy body, the diet must contain adequate amounts of vitamins and minerals, otherwise deficiency diseases can occur.

Calcium and *Vitamin D* are needed to build strong bones and teeth. A deficiency disease called rickets will occur if either or both these substances are lacking. Rickets is the softening of bones and can be seen in deformed (not straight) leg bones.

Iron is needed for the formation of red blood cells. Anaemia results if iron is deficient in the diet.

Iodine forms part of the hormone thyroxine (see section on Endocrines, page 156).

Vitamin A is required for healthy eyes, or night blindness may result.

Lack of *Vitamin C* causes bleeding gums (scurvy) and slow healing of wounds.

Lack of the *B group* of vitamins results in a range of deficiency diseases.

Activity 3

5 Name a rich food source for each of the above vitamins and minerals.

THE EXCRETORY SYSTEM

This consists of the kidneys, tubes (ureter) leading to the bladder where urine is stored, and a tube through which the liquid waste exits the body (urethra). The functions of the kidneys are to remove the waste products of protein metabolism and excess water from the body, and also to regulate the chemical composition of the blood.

When the bladder is full of urine, it sends

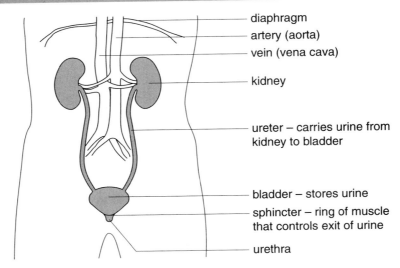

Figure 5.9   *The excretory system*

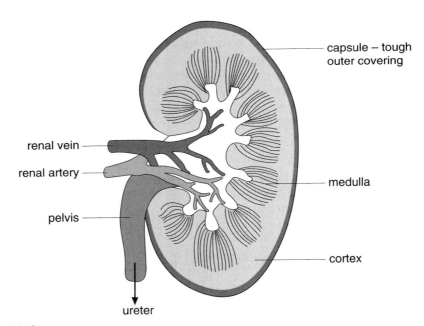

Figure 5.10   *A kidney*

a message to the brain. The brain responds by sending a message to the muscles surrounding the exit to the bladder, they relax and the bladder is emptied.

THE NERVOUS SYSTEM

This consists of two linking parts:

1 the central nervous system made up of the

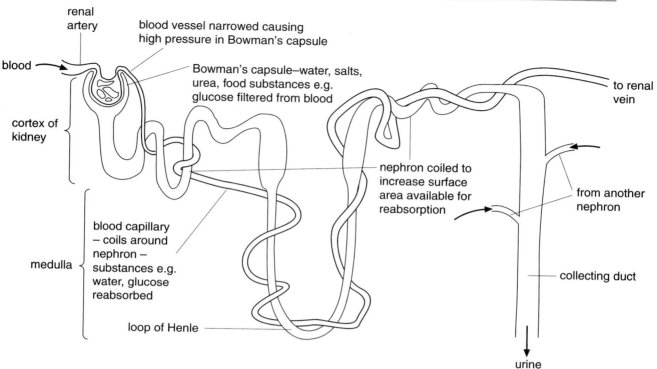

Figure 5.11   *A nephron*

brain and spinal cord

2 peripheral nerve fibres. Sensory nerves carry messages from the sense organs to the central nervous system, and motor nerves carry the response from the central nervous system to muscles and glands.

Because of their specialised functions (conducting electrical impulses) nerve cells have a different shape from the cells described earlier in the chapter (see page 146).

- Neurones never touch.
- The gap between neurones is called a synapse.
- An impulse crosses the gap using chemical transmitters, e.g. acetylcholine.

Note: nerve impulses pass in *one* direction only.

The nervous system controls the activities of the body, and makes sure they all work

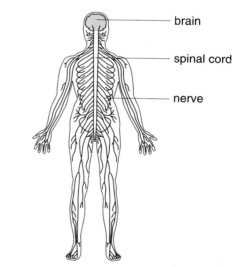

Figure 5.12   *The nervous system*

together efficiently. Specialised parts of the brain are involved in:

1 interpreting signals from the sense organs,

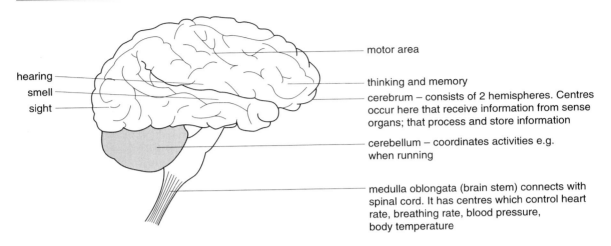

Figure 5.13   *The brain*

e.g. interpreting speech and other sounds, sight, touch, etc.

2 regulating activities that a person has no conscious control over, e.g. heart beat, body temperature, etc.

3 using information received from sense organs and muscles to maintain balance and coordinate activities such as walking, jumping, and hopping.

Reflex actions are those which happen very quickly in response to a stimulus; e.g. if you step on a sharp stone in bare feet, the foot is immediately pulled away

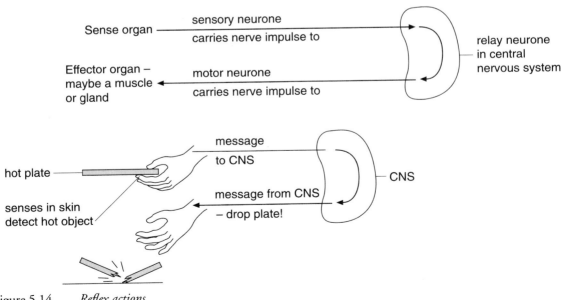

Figure 5.14   *Reflex actions*

THE REPRODUCTIVE SYSTEM

Reproduction can take place in two ways:

1 asexually: in simple organisms, reproduction takes places with just one organism. The offspring has the same genetic makeup as the parent; e.g. bacteria reproduce by splitting into two identical bacteria.

2 sexually: two organisms are needed: a male and female organism of the same species. When fertilisation takes place, the nuclei of the two cells fuse together, forming a *zygote*.

In humans, men produce sperm, and women produce ova (eggs). After fertilisation, the zygote implants into the prepared lining of the uterus, and develops into a baby.

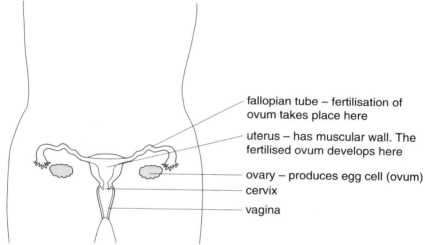

fallopian tube – fertilisation of ovum takes place here

uterus – has muscular wall. The fertilised ovum develops here

ovary – produces egg cell (ovum)

cervix

vagina

Figure 5.15   *The female reproductive organs*

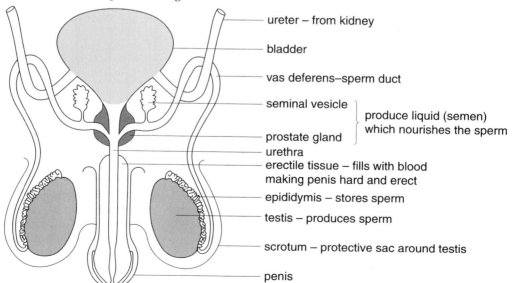

ureter – from kidney

bladder

vas deferens–sperm duct

seminal vesicle ⎫
                 ⎬ produce liquid (semen)
prostate gland ⎭ which nourishes the sperm

urethra

erectile tissue – fills with blood making penis hard and erect

epididymis – stores sperm

testis – produces sperm

scrotum – protective sac around testis

penis

Figure 5.16   *The male reproductive organs*

Table 5.1   The Endocrine Glands, their major hormones and effects

Gland	Hormone	Effect
Pituitary	Trophic hormones	Cause other endocrines to produce their hormones; e.g. the thyroid to produce thyroxine
	Growth hormone	Controls the growth of the body. Too much causes excessive growth, too little causes dwarfism
	Oxytocin	Secreted during childbirth, makes the uterus contract
Gonads:		
Ovaries	Oestrogen	Stimulates development of secondary female sexual characteristics during puberty and prepares the uterus to receive a fertilised ovum
	Progesterone	Involved with oestrogen in control of menstrual cycle
Testes	Testosterone	Produces secondary male characteristics
Adrenal	Adrenaline	Produced in response to stress to prepare the body for action
Thyroid	Thyroxine	Controls the rate of metabolism of the body
Pancreas	Insulin	Controls the level of blood glucose by stimulating body cells to take it in. People suffer from diabetes when too little insulin in produced, so that blood glucose rises to levels that can be life-threatening.

In women, an egg is produced every month at approximately the middle of the menstrual cycle. If it is not fertilised, it exits the body with the now redundant uterus lining; this is commonly called the *period.*

Genetic information contained in the nucleus of the sperm and ovum, is passed onto the next generation. The baby will therefore have a combination of characteristics from both father and mother.

THE ENDOCRINE SYSTEM

This consists of glands situated around the body, that produce powerful chemical messengers called *hormones.* The endocrine glands are unlike other glands (e.g. the salivary glands in the mouth) in that they do

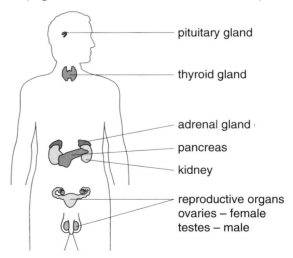

pituitary gland

thyroid gland

adrenal gland

pancreas

kidney

reproductive organs
ovaries – female
testes – male

Figure 5.17   *The endocrine system*

not have a duct along which their secretions pass to the particular area where they work. Hormones are secreted directly into the blood stream: this carries them to the target organ which responds to them.

The *Pituitary* gland is situated at the base of the brain, and can be considered the controlling influence of many of the other endocrines. It is sometimes called the 'master' gland. It secretes hormones which stimulate other endocrines to produce more of their hormones, e.g. it stimulates the thyroid gland to produce more thyroxine.

THE MUSCULO-SKELETAL SYSTEM

The skeleton consists of 206 bones of different shapes and sizes, which have three functions:

1 support of the body
2 protection of vital organs, e.g. the rib cage protects the lungs and heart
3 movement. Where bones meet, they form joints that with the aid of muscles, create movement

Activity 4

6 Can you think of another organ that is protected by bone?
7 Almost all bones meet to form movable joints. Can you think of some joints where movement does not occur?

Bones

Although they are hard, bones are made up of living cells. Otherwise, when a bone breaks, it would not be able to mend itself. The cells are surrounded by minerals, mostly calcium salts, that give strength and rigidity to the bone. Bone cells are like any others,

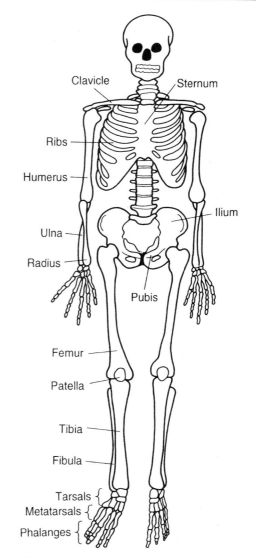

Figure 5.18   *The skeleton*

and receive nourishment via the blood supply. Specialist areas in some bones are concerned with the formation of red and white blood cells i.e. the pelvis, and in long bones such as the femur.

Long bones have two rounded heads at either end of the long shaft. The heads are covered with cartilage. At joints, bones are held together by tough rope-like structures called ligaments.

(a) Sliding joint e.g. between the vertebrae

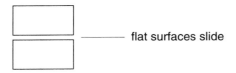

flat surfaces slide

(b) Ball and socket e.g. at shoulder

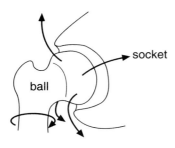

socket

ball

(c) Hinge joint e.g. knee

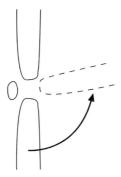

Figure 5.19   *Different types of joint*

Ball and socket, and hinge joints are constructed in a special way with *synovial* fluid between the bones. This reduces the amount of friction between the bones (see page 170).

Muscles

Muscles are attached to bones by fibres called *tendons*. When muscles contract they pull on the tendon, which pulls the bone, and movement results. Many muscles work in pairs: as one contracts, the other relaxes and vice versa. An example of this is in the arm: see Fig. 5.21.

Activity 5

8 Can you think of another example of:
a a hinge joint?
b a ball and socket joint?

Muscle tissue has a special function; it can contract (get smaller), and relax (become longer again). A lot of energy is needed by the muscles to perform this special function, and it is obtained from the chemical reaction of oxygen with glucose within the muscle cells. They therefore have a very efficient network of blood capillaries and nerve fibres running between them.

There are three types of muscle tissue in the body. They have different structures for their different jobs:

1 *Voluntary* muscles — these are attached to the skeleton and can be contracted and relaxed at will.
2 *Involuntary* muscle — is controlled by the central nervous system e.g. the muscles in the alimentary canal responsible for peristalsis.
3 *Cardiac* muscle found only in the heart, and specially adapted for continuous action.

Summary

Organ systems work together:

- The digestive system needs the circulatory system to carry the products of digestion to the body cells.
- The respiratory system uses the circulatory system, because the red blood cells carry the oxygen and carbon dioxide from the cells to the lungs.

For the body to work efficiently, the environment inside it needs to be stable.

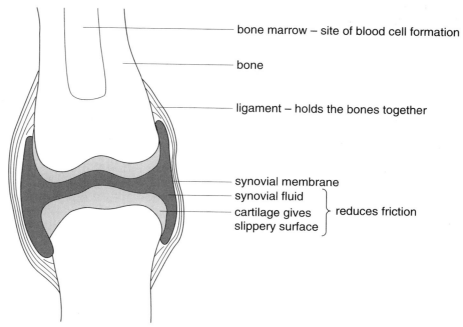

bone marrow – site of blood cell formation

bone

ligament – holds the bones together

synovial membrane
synovial fluid
cartilage gives
slippery surface } reduces friction

Figure 5.20   *The structure of a synovial joint*

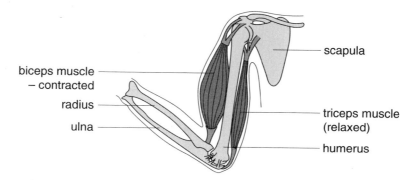

biceps muscle
– contracted

radius

ulna

scapula

triceps muscle
(relaxed)

humerus

Figure 5.21   *Muscles in the arm*

Therefore conditions need to be monitored constantly and adjustments made if necessary. This process is called *homeostasis*. Many organs are involved in homeostasis.

Activity 6

9 Name other systems that work together.

10 Can you name the organs that are involved in homeostasis in the body?

Observation and measurement

Observation and the taking of measurements of a person can help in many ways:

- to help in assessing health and disease
- as an aid to diagnosis of disease
- to monitor changes
- to monitor growth and development

Observations and measurements can be made in many different settings e.g. day centres, hospitals, baby clinics, residential care, etc. We can also use observation and measurement in our homes in assessing our own and our family's health.

In the different settings, we can use many different observations and measurements.

Activity 7

 11 What observations and/or measurements do you think would be used in:

a a baby clinic
b a residential home for elderly people?

You should be able to see from the above exercise that we need to know what to look for and measure, with different people in different settings.

OBSERVATIONS

Posture

The way a person holds themselves can tell us much about how they feel:

- If a person is walking with energy, head up, eyes focused on their surroundings, they will be feeling confident.

- When a person is feeling 'down' or upset, they are more likely to be walking slowly, looking down, with shoulders hunched (see Fig. 4.3, on page 122).

Good posture is important in order to prevent problems such as backache after lifting or standing for long periods of time. Constant bad posture during growth may lead to round shoulders and stooping in later life, which may result in breathing difficulties.

Skin and complexion

The skin is an important organ of the body, and has many functions, such as temperature control (see page 162), and it is a vital barrier to the entry of micro-organisms.

The colour of the skin can be observed:

1 on the *face* – are the cheeks flushed and red? If so this could indicate that the person is too warm or has a high body temperature.
   i *pallor* (lack of colour) may mean a low body temperature, or that a person is cold or in shock.
   ii *cyanosis* (blue colour) of the lips and skin may indicate that the blood is not carrying enough oxygen, possibly because of problems with the lungs (e.g. bronchitis), or the circulation (purple fingers and toes can be caused by cold).

2 on the *body* – constant bumps and bruises could mean either that a person is having difficulty with balance, or is bumping into things because of not being able to see clearly.

The texture of the skin can vary from greasy

to very dry. Excessive dryness can result in cracks in the skin where bacteria and other micro-organisms enter and cause infection.

The feet and nails

Observation of the feet may show that a person has corns caused by badly fitting shoes. People who have mobility problems sometimes have difficulty cutting their toe nails, and drying between their toes after bathing. The services of a chiropodist may be needed.

The hair

To keep hair in good condition, it needs washing and brushing regularly. School children's hair will need inspecting as they are at risk of lice infestation. Lice cannot jump or fly, but they crawl onto other heads when they touch.

Nits (the eggs), are seen as small white blobs on hair close to the scalp, in the neck region and around the ears. When the louse hatches, it feeds on blood from the scalp. This causes irritation and scratching. Lotions to kill both lice and eggs are available at the chemist or baby clinic. Prevention is better than cure however, and combing the hair every night using a fine-toothed comb is the best method.

The eyes

The eyes should be clear and alert, with no discolouration of the whites. If a person is suffering from jaundice because of liver disease, the white of the eye becomes yellow. Infections of the eye like conjunctivitis causes redness and abnormal secretions.

Levels of consciousness

We use many words and phrases to describe levels of consciousness e.g. lethargic, 'not with it', confused, unconscious. These words refer to both the physical and mental states, and the meaning of the words is not always clear: e.g. 'unconscious' is generally used to describe when someone cannot be roused after being knocked out, but it also means to be unaware, so it can also be used to describe ordinary sleep.

The different levels of consciousness can be listed as:

1 totally alert, physically and mentally awake
2 alert physically, but mentally confused; able to cope on a physical level, but not able to answer questions in a lucid way. This can be a transient state in some people, but in others it can be an indication of the onset of some disease
3 semi-conscious: person is almost 'asleep', but will respond to a painful stimulus
4 unconscious: person cannot be roused, but the pupils of the eye will respond to light. If the pupils will not respond to light, this may be an indication of brain damage

The Glasgow Coma Scale is used in hospitals to assess levels of consciousness. The scale is in three parts: eye-opening assessment, verbal response and motor response.

Mood

Everyone has days when they feel wonderful, and life is great. On other days problems may occur and we feel less good, and less able to cope. These mood swings are normal. Occasionally however a person may become clinically depressed. This may be recognised by:

- a person having difficulty sleeping
- eating disorders, either compulsive eating, bingeing, or eating very little
- a lack of interest in their appearance, or in life

- lethargy
- difficulty in concentrating

Everyone suffers from one or more of the above at times, so it is very difficult to assess whether a person is just feeling 'down', or is in need of specialist help and support.

MEASUREMENTS

Measurements of any kind need to be taken with accuracy. This means that we need to be familiar with any instrument used to take measurements with, be it a ruler to measure height, or a thermometer to take temperature.

We also need to be able to relate any measurement to a table or graph which will tell us whether the result is 'normal' or not.

Height and weight

Measurement of weight and height in babies can give an indication of their continuing development. It is regularly done in health centres and baby clinics throughout the country. A baby will have a height/weight chart.

Three lines are shown for both height and weight. These lines are the result of research of the subject in many hundreds of babies, and are described as *percentiles*. The middle lines are the average or 50th percentile. The top and bottom lines are the 10th and 90th percentiles respectively. They mean that 10 per cent of the results will lie outside each of these lines, so that 10 per cent of babies will be bigger than the 90th percentile, and 10 per cent of babies will be smaller than the 10th percentile. Results can therefore lie outside the 10th and 90th percentile and still be considered normal. Different charts are used for boys and girls.

Obesity, or being overweight for your height, can increase the risk of heart disease,

strokes etc. So here again we can use a graph or table to assess if our height matches our weight. Loss of height with ageing may indicate the development of osteoporosis (loss of bone density and strength), especially in women after the menopause.

Body temperature

This is measured using a clinical thermometer. Thermometers work on the principle that substances expand on heating, and contract on cooling. So that we can read a clinical thermometer, a constriction is put in the tube which stops the liquid contracting back down the tube. After reading, the thermometer has to be shaken to allow the liquid to be returned to the bulb, before it can be used again.

Activity 8

 12 What is normal body temperature?

In hospitals, thermometers have to be disinfected after use to prevent transmission of disease.

A plastic strip that changes colour with different temperatures is now replacing the clinical thermometer. The strip is held firmly to the forehead for half a minute, and then the temperature is read off the scale.

Increase in temperature can indicate infection (see page 165).

Pulse and breathing rates

Pulse rate is the rate at which the heart beats. It can be counted at sites in the neck, wrist, foot and groin, and is caused by the 'pulse' of blood that is pushed out of the left ventricle of the heart along the arteries. The pulse rate in babies can be as high as 160 beats per minute. This falls to below 80 beats per minute by the age of seven years when the body is at rest.

Breathing rate is the number of breaths taken in 1 minute, and is usually between 8 and 12.

Increase in activity will result in a rise in both pulse and breathing rates. This is to increase the amount of glucose and oxygen available to the body cells for conversion to energy. A trained athlete's pulse may rise to nearly 200 beats per minute. This could be dangerous in an unfit person.

Activity 9

Take and record your pulse.
Run on the spot or do some other activity for one minute, and take your pulse again. Take it every minute until the rate returns to your resting rate.

- Compare your results with others in your class.
- Repeat the above for breathing rate.
- What conclusions can you make about your own results and those of your class?

Pulse rate and breathing rate can be linked. Disturbances of pulse rate caused by heart disease will cause changes in breathing rate.

On the other hand, changes in breathing rate resulting from respiratory disease can cause a change in pulse rate. Intense pain will cause a rise in both rates.

Measurements taken to assess lung function

The volume of air taken into the lungs with each breath is called the *tidal volume*, and in an adult it is about half a litre. We can increase the tidal volume during exercise, so it is clear that the lungs are not fully inflated or deflated when the body is at rest. We have a lot of lung capacity in reserve.

If we breath in as far as possible, and then out as far as possible, this volume is known as the *vital capacity*. In healthy adults this volume is approximately four litres. People suffering from bronchitis or asthma may have a reduced vital capacity.

When we have emptied our lungs as much as we can, there is still some air remaining, because the lungs are not completely deflated. The volume remaining is called the *residual volume*, and is about one litre.

Measurement of these volumes is made using an instrument called a spirometer.

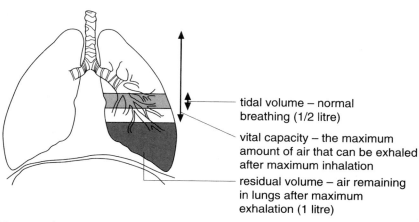

tidal volume – normal breathing (1/2 litre)

vital capacity – the maximum amount of air that can be exhaled after maximum inhalation

residual volume – air remaining in lungs after maximum exhalation (1 litre)

Figure 5.22   *Measuring lung capacity*

Fluid input and output measurements

The fluid balance of the body in health is regulated by the kidneys. Imbalance of fluid can be seen by its build up in the tissues (oedema), especially in the feet. It may indicate renal or circulatory problems.

In hospitals and other care establishments, charts are used routinely for recording a person's temperature, pulse and breathing rates. Fluid balance charts to record fluid consumed and urine excreted are also used when necessary.

Activity 10

Keep a fluid input and output diary for yourself over two days. Note times and quantities of fluid you drink, and the times and quantities of urine you pass.

Design a chart which will effectively record the results.

Note: input does not equal output. This is because water is lost from the body in other ways and places.

13 Name at least two ways that fluid is lost from the body, other than by *micturition* (passage of urine).

14 We obtain fluid in more ways than just drinking. Can you name them?

In hot weather, more water is lost as sweat in order to cool the body (see page 166). Urine output will be decreased, and we will become thirsty and so drink more to maintain the fluid balance in the body.

If kidney function fails, or if the kidney becomes infected, less urine will be excreted, and so fluid and wastes of metabolism will accumulate in the body.

Another measurement very often taken is that of *blood pressure*, which measures the pressure exerted when the heart contracts and when it relaxes: see page 173, Hypertension.

Summary

Consider all that we have looked at in this section, and then decide what being 'healthy' really means.

- Does it mean being disease free?
- Is a person healthy who is physically well but mentally depressed?

As you can see, we need to be both physically and mentally well to be termed healthy.

It involves all our physical and mental processes working together to create what we really mean by a *healthy* person.

As health care professionals, we need to always consider *total care* of people, and not focus purely on the physical or mental signs.

Applying science to care contexts

In this section we will look at how science can be applied in a care setting; e.g.:

- how we can make sure that a person is comfortable, neither too hot nor too cold

- how we can reduce the problems caused by friction and pressure
- how we can make use of levers to make lifting easier.

Body temperature and its measurement

When you get a bottle of milk out of the refrigerator, the hand holding the milk feels cold because it is losing heat to the cold bottle in an attempt to make the temperatures equal. In the same way, a warm person loses heat to a cold room. Long-term exposure to cold may result in lowering of body temperature or *hypothermia*.

Air is a good insulator, and by wearing several layers of clothes, the person will be insulated from the cold by the layers of air between them. Windows are double glazed for the same reason.

Comment

ⓘ Body temperature does vary throughout 24 hours by up to a half of a degree. It is lowest at 4 am. If body temperature rises above normal, we suffer from *pyrexia*. A fall below normal is termed *hypothermia*.

Before we look at factors that can affect body temperature, we need to understand how heat is transferred.

Transferring heat

There are three ways in which heat can be passed on:

1 *Radiation* This is the heat given off by any hot object, either the sun (our ulti-

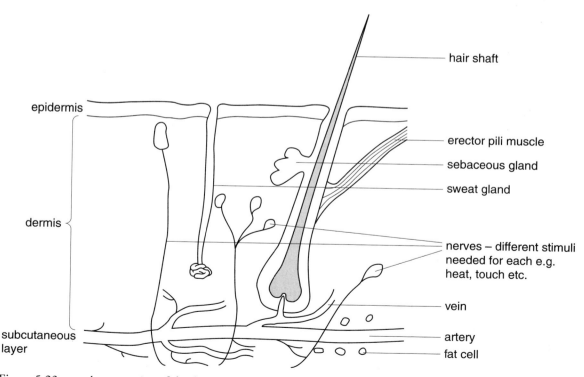

Figure 5.23   *A cross-section of the skin*

mate source of heat), a fire or ourselves. It travels in straight lines as heat rays, and it can travel through a vacuum.

2 *Convection* This is heat flow through a gas or liquid. When a gas or liquid is heated, it increases in volume and so its density decreases. The hot gas or liquid will therefore rise, be cooled and fall. In this way a convection current is formed.

3 *Conduction* This occurs in solids when heat is passed from particle to particle. It happens rapidly in metals, and these are called good conductors. Substances such as cork, air, and wool do not conduct heat and are termed good insulators. Heat produced by friction is passed by conduction through the skin when cold fingers or toes are rubbed.

THE SKIN

The skin is the body's largest organ. It protects the body from bacterial attack, and helps regulate the temperature of the body. During exercise heat energy is produced rapidly in the muscles: see Fig. 5.23.

Activity 11

 15 What do cells need to produce energy?

16 Write the equation to show how energy is produced.

To keep body temperature constant, heat can be lost in the following ways:

1 Sweating: when sweat evaporates, it takes the heat it needs to do so from the body, therefore having a cooling effect.

2 The body becomes 'flushed'. Blood vessels dilate (get larger) near the surface of the skin, so more heat can be lost.

3 Heat is lost by the body when eliminating waste, e.g. warm urine and faeces.

In cold weather, the metabolism of the body speeds up and this results in an increase in heat production to keep the body temperature constant: therefore more food will be needed by the body. Blood vessels constrict (become smaller), to reduce the amount of heat lost through the skin, and the skin may appear purple. Shivering, which is a jerky muscular movement, is used to increase heat production. 'Goose pimples' are produced on the skin by the erecti pili muscles contracting and pulling the hair follicle upright. This pushes the skin into the characteristic 'pimples'. The raised hairs attempt to trap a layer of air next to the body to insulate it, and lessen heat loss. How effective this is in people with very little body hair is questionable!

In order to keep the temperature of the body constant, the body has to balance all these mechanisms.

Heat production	Heat loss
by all cells in the body, especially those in the liver and muscles	• by elimination of waste • by evaporation of sweat • from blood vessels through the skin

Activity 12

 17 When visiting an elderly person in their own home, what signs would make you suspect the person was suffering from hypothermia?

18 What could you do to warm someone who has hypothermia?

19 What advice could you give a person about keeping warm?

20 What could you do to reduce a child's high temperature?

COMMENT

ⓘ Vigorous exercise produces a lot of heat within the muscles, and this may cause a slight rise in body temperature. Pyrexia (increase in body temperature) can also be a way that the body responds to infection (being attacked by microbes).

Pyrexia helps the body's response to infection, but it also causes discomfort, e.g. headache, sweating, loss of appetite, etc. Excessive rises in body temperature can result in convulsions and other medical complications.

When the skin temperature is 33 °C, a person feels comfortable, neither hot nor cold. The amount of water (humidity) in the atmosphere will also affect whether a person feels comfortable or not. When there is high humidity, sweat on the skin cannot evaporate easily, so less heat is lost.

Heat regulation in babies is not well developed, so it is important that they sleep in a warm room in winter. On a warm summer's day they should wear loose, cotton clothing, and be kept out of direct sunlight.

FOOD AND ENERGY

Food chains

The energy we need to stay alive, to work and play comes from the food we eat.

Green plants can make their own food from carbon dioxide and water, in a process called *photosynthesis*. During this process, energy from the sun is used in the green leaves to combine 6 molecules of carbon dioxide and 6 molecules of water into simple sugars like glucose, and oxygen. Glucose can then be made into other food substances e.g. starch, proteins.

$$6CO_2 \ + \ \overset{\text{many}}{\underset{\text{stages}}{6H_2O}} \ \rightarrow \ C_6H_{12}O_6 + \ 6O_2$$

carbon dioxide   water   glucose oxygen

Green plants are called *producers* and the organisms which rely on them for food are *consumers*.

sun
↓

producer   green plants
                e.g. grass
                ↓

primary   sheep
consumer   a *herbivore*, eats only plants
                ↓

secondary   man
consumer   a secondary consumer can be a *carnivore* eating only meat, or like man, an *omnivore* eating both plants and animals

Figure 5.25   *A food chain*

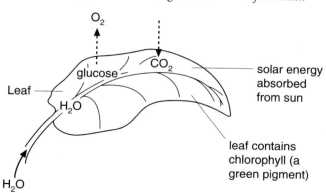

Figure 5.24   *A food web*

Another example of a food chain is:

green plants → rabbit → fox
e.g. carrot

But rabbits eat other plants as well as carrots, and foxes eat birds and frogs in addition to rabbits. So instead of a simple food chain we can draw a *food web*.

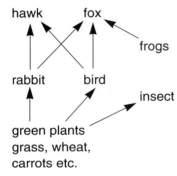

Figure 5.26   *A food web*

If changes occur in the population of any member of a food web, it will affect every other member in the web, i.e. they are all *dependent* on each other.

Energy is usually measured in *joules* or *kilojoules*, and sometimes in *calories* or *kilocalories*. To convert calories to joules, multiply the calorie by 4.2:

1 calorie = 4.2 joules

When we look at a food chain, we are actually looking at how energy is passed from organism to organism, and how each organism makes use of that energy.

Because every organism uses energy during respiration, and loses some energy in waste products that are excreted, less energy is available for the next organism in the chain. Ninety per cent of energy is used or lost in waste, and only 10 per cent is actually passed on.

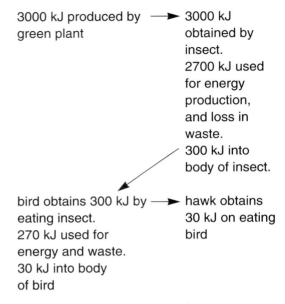

Figure 5.27   *Energy loss in a food chain*

This loss of energy along a food chain will mean that there will be a limit to the number of consumers in a food chain. We are primary or secondary consumers in most food chains.

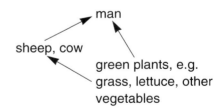

Figure 5.28   *Food chain including man*

Short food chains are therefore more appropriate in developing countries when large numbers of people need to be fed efficiently.

As we pass along a food chain, the size of the organisms gets larger, but their numbers become less. This can be shown in a *pyramid of biomass*.

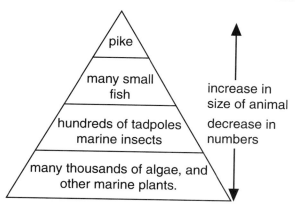

Figure 5.29   *A pyramid of biomass*

Adenosine Triphosphate and energy in the body

$$glucose + oxygen \rightarrow \frac{carbon}{dioxode} + water + energy$$
(many stages)

During respiration, the energy released is not in a form that can be used by the body. The energy is used to make a compound called *adenosine triphosphate (ATP)*.

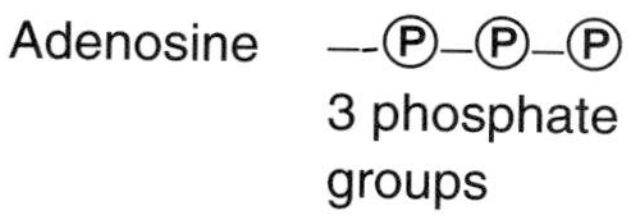

Adenosine   —(P)–(P)–(P)
3 phosphate
groups

Figure 5.30   *Structure of ATP*

When ATP breaks down, forming adenosine diphosphate and a phosphate group, a lot of energy is released that can be used by the cells of the body

$$ATP \rightarrow ADP + P + Energy$$

ATP acts as a holding mechanism or short-term energy store. When energy is needed by the body cells, ATP is rapidly broken down as shown above, and energy is released. Use of ATP as a holding molecule means that:

• energy can be released rapidly when it is needed, e.g. when doing strenuous exercise
• energy is always available
• energy is produced in a controlled manner, so none is wasted.

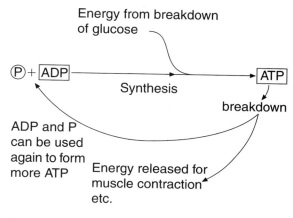

Figure 5.31   *Use of ATP*

Energy is needed by the body for many reasons e.g.

• to keep vital organs working
• to maintain body temperature
• to build and repair cells
• for muscle contraction
• for passage of nerve impulses
• in pregnant women to build the baby's body, and after birth, to make milk for the baby.

Individuals will have different requirements for energy depending on:

• age
• sex
• occupation
• the kind of hobbies
• the state of the body.

You know from Chapter 1 that individuals have differing requirements for nutrients as well as for energy.

FRICTION

Rubbing hands together when they are cold, will make them warmer because of the heat created by *friction*.

Friction can cause pressure sores in people who are bed-ridden. At risk are those areas which are in contact with the bed clothes e.g. the buttocks, heels, etc. Creams and talcum powder applied to the skin can reduce friction and help prevent pressure sores occurring. The use of special cushions, air (ripple) and water beds and sheepskins can also help.

Turning people onto one side and then the other can help to alleviate pressure sores, but care needs to be taken when lifting or turning people, or helping them to stand so as not to cause pain by friction or the pressure of the hands. Some people may bruise easily especially older people.

Hypodermic needles used to give injections or take blood cause pain because of penetrating the skin, and also because of the friction or drag on the skin as the needle passes through it. Very fine bore needles with a smooth, shiny surface reduce the friction and hence the pain felt.

Friction can be reduced by:

- lubricating the surfaces with oils, creams, etc.
- having smooth shiny surfaces
- reducing the area of the surfaces in contact by using ball bearings for example.

Activity 13

 21 Can you think of one area in the body considered in section 1 of this chapter, which makes use of two of these methods to reduce friction?

Mucus is another natural lubricant of the body.

Low friction materials are required at other times during caring:

- a shiny plastic tube is used in catheterisation
- hip and other joints for replacement are made of shiny metals

Uses of friction

We have looked at ways to reduce friction because of its effects, but friction is useful in many ways. We could not walk without friction between the feet and the ground. Think what happens if we try to walk on ice!

- A car has a rough tyre tread to increase friction, and promote road-holding, but it will still skid on ice or when the road surface is very wet.
- Writing on paper would be impossible without friction between pen and paper.

EFFECTS OF PRESSURE

Pressure is a *force*. It tells us how concentrated a force is; e.g. the pressure created on a floor by a woman wearing flat heeled shoes is less than by the same woman in stiletto heels. Pressure depends on the surface area on which the force is applied.

Another example is pushing a drawing pin into a notice-board with a thumb. It goes in easily, but if you used the same force to push your thumb into the notice-board, it will not go in at all.

The force of gravity pulls a liquid down into its container, causing pressure on all sides of the container, and also on any object put into the water. A boat floats, because of the upward force of the water. A person in water experiences the same force, and it gives

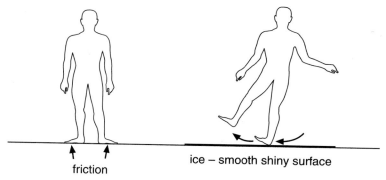

friction   ice – smooth shiny surface

Figure 5.32   *The effects of friction*

a degree of what is called **buoyancy**. Exercising or swimming in water reduces the pressure on joints, and can help people with arthritis or those recovering from serious injury to bones and joints.

Pressure can also cause changes in shape. Think what happens if you squeeze a rubber ball. As discussed already it is necessary to take care when lifting a person, so damage is not done to skin, joints and bones. With ageing, bone density and hence bone strength, diminishes. It has been known for bones to be broken through careless lifting.

Pressure is created by blood in the arteries of the body by the heart beating. If the arteries become furred up by fatty deposits, this will increase blood pressure. Ageing causes the walls or the arteries to become less elastic, and again blood pressure rises. Some people have significantly raised blood pressure and suffer from **hypertension**. These people are more likely to have strokes.

As discussed earlier, the cranium protects the brain from damage caused by knocks etc. However, a severe blow to the head will cause bruising and in some cases swelling of the brain tissue. If this happens, the pressure inside the cranium will rise. Other conditions e.g. cerebral haemorrhage will also increase inter-cranial pressure. As the pressure rises, it depresses the activities of the

brain, and eventually may cause coma. Medication, and sometimes an operation, will be necessary to lower the inter-cranial pressure.

LEVERS

The raising of the arm as seen in the section on the skeleton, is an example of a lever. Knowledge of how levers work can help us lift objects more easily.

Three points on a lever can be identified:

- the force needed to move an object is the *effort*

- the weight which is to be moved is the *load*

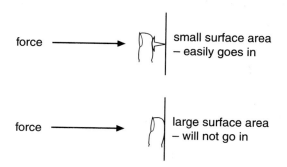

force →   small surface area – easily goes in

force →   large surface area – will not go in

Figure 5.33   *The effect of pressure on different sized surface areas*

- the point at which the lever pivots (turns) is the *fulcrum*.

There are three types or orders of lever, depending on the arrangement of the effort, load and fulcrum: see Figures 5.34, 5.35 and 5.36. In the body the effort is applied by muscles.

Summary

This chapter has shown how we can turn to science to explain how our bodies work. By using scientific knowledge and making critical observations and measurements, we can understand and treat unusual human behaviour, and determine whether bodily functions are working as efficiently and effectively as they can.

Health has been linked here both to physical and mental processes. As health and social care professionals, we need to consider both elements when treating another person.

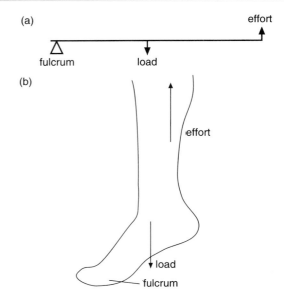

Figure 5.35   *Second-class levers: (a) the principle; (b) a foot*

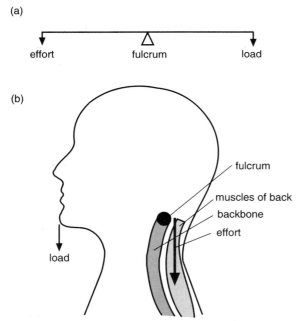

Figure 5.34   *First-class levers: (a) the principle; (b) a human head*

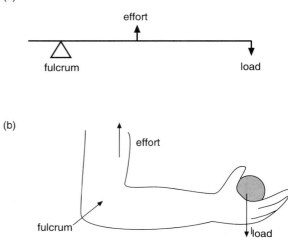

Figure 5.36   *Third-class levers: (a) the principle; (b) an arm*

DEFINITIONS

alveoli structures like bunches of grapes at the end of bronchioles in lungs where exchange of gases occurs

artery blood vessel carrying blood away from the heart

assimilation absorption and use of food by body cells

atria upper chambers of the heart (plural atrium)

bile formed in liver, stored in gall bladder, helps digestion of fats

central nervous system (CNS) consists of brain and spinal cord

conduction passage of heat from particle to particle in a solid

consumer organism in a food chain which survive by eating the other organisms in the chain

convection heat transfer in liquids and gases

diabetes disease where too little insulin is produced by the pancreas so blood glucose levels are high

diaphragm muscle separating thorax from abdomen, involved in breathing movements

diastolic pressure blood pressure when heart is relaxed

diffusion movement of molecules from a region of high concentration to a region of low concentration

duct tube along which liquids flow

endocrine gland a ductless gland, produces chemical messengers called hormones

epididymis tube where sperm are stored

excretion removal of waste from the body

fallopian tube tube from ovary to uterus. Fertilisation of ovum by a sperm takes place here

food chain the series of organisms, beginning with producers, through which energy is passed

friction resistance caused when two surfaces rub together

homeostasis maintenance of stable conditions within the body

hormone chemical messenger produced by the endocrine glands

hypertension high blood pressure

hypothermia low body temperature

insulin hormone produced by the pancreas which controls blood glucose levels

intercostal muscle between the ribs, responsible with the diaphragm for breathing movement

ligament holds bones together

metabolism the chemical reactions that a cell needs to perform to release energy, grow, etc.

nerve impulse the chemical and electrical changes passing along a nerve produced by a stimulus

neurone nerve cells which conduct nerve impulses

nucleus part of cell that contains genetic information

oesophagus food tube from the mouth to the stomach

organ group of tissues organised for a task e.g. heart

ovary female reproductive organ which produces ova

peristalsis wave of contraction in alimentary canal which moves food along

producer green plants which make food from carbon dioxide and water using energy from the sun

pulmonary circulation circulation of deoxygenated blood from heart to lungs

pyrexia high body temperature

reflex rapid response occurring without thought

residual volume after forced exhalation, this is the amount of air remaining in the lungs

respiration chemical reactions taking place in the cell which release energy

sebaceous gland   attached to hair follicle, produces sebum

sebum   greasy liquid from the sebaceous gland, keeps skin supple, waterproof and is an antiseptic

sensory neurone   nerve from sense organs to C.N.S.

spinal cord   nerve fibres from brain extending down the body inside the protective vertebral column

systemic circulation   circulation of blood to all body cells except in lungs

systolic pressure   pressure of heart on contraction

sphygmomanometer   instrument for measuring blood pressure

testes   male reproductive organs which produce sperm

thyroid gland   endocrine gland which produces thyroxine

tidal volume   volume of air entering and leaving the lungs at rest

trachea   windpipe

tendon   attaches bone to muscle

urea   waste product of protein metabolism, excreted by the kidneys

ureter   carries urine from kidney to bladder

urethra   tube carrying urine from bladder to outside body

uterus   (womb) organ where a baby develops

tissue   specialised body cells grouped to perform a task

vein   blood vessel carrying blood to heart

ventricles   lower chambers of the heart

villi   projections into the small intestine, increase the surface area for absorption of soluble food particles

vital capacity   after inhaling as far as possible, this is the maximum amount of air that can be exhaled

ANSWERS TO QUESTIONS

Activity 1

1 The alveoli increase the surface area available for exchange of gases.

2 The amount of oxygen will be reduced, and carbon dioxide will increase.

Activity 2

3 The ventricles have thicker walls because they need to push the blood to the lungs and around the rest of the body.

4 A valve prevents back-flow of blood.

Activity 3

5 *Calcium*   dairy foods, e.g. milk cheese
Vitamin A   fish liver oils, margarine
Iron   liver, chocolate
Iodine   sea foods, salt
Vitamin A   dairy foods, fish liver oils, carrots
Vitamin C   blackcurrants, green peppers
Vitamin B   cereals, meat

Activity 4

6 The cranium protects the brain.

7 There is no movement between the bones of the cranium.

Activity 5

8 a hinge joint: fingers
   b ball and socket joint: shoulder joint

Activity 6

9 The excretory system works with the circulatory system.

10 Kidney, lungs and liver are involved in homeostasis in the body.

Activity 7

11 a height and weight measurements, hearing tests, observation of development
  b observations of all types of behaviour

Activity 8

12 37° C

Activity 10

13 Fluid is lost when the body is sweating, and is lost as water vapour when breathing out.
14 We obtain water from food, and we make water during metabolism.

Activity 11

15 Cells need food in the form of glucose and oxygen to produce energy.

16 food + oxygen → carbon dioxide + water + energy

Activity 12

17 Signs of hypothermia include: cold room, skin cold to touch and pale, lethargy.
18 To warm someone with hypothermia, wrap in blanket, give warm (not hot) drink.
19 To keep warm, wear many layers of clothes plus a hat and gloves, move around, take regular hot food and drink.
20 You can reduce a child's temperature by giving him or her cool drinks, removing clothing, giving paracetamol by mouth, and giving a sponge bath.

Activity 13

21 Synovial joint (see pages 157–59).

6

MEETING THE NEEDS OF INDIVIDUALS IN DIFFERENT CARE SETTINGS

AIMS AND OBJECTIVES

The aim of this chapter is to enable you to understand what is involved in meeting the needs of people who are cared for by others.

At the end of this chapter you should be able to:

• summarise the assessment methods used to assess individual need in care settings

• describe how care plans are used in meeting individual care needs

• explore individual needs in the care setting, and how they are met

• investigate factors that influence the delivery of care in different settings

---

Assessing individual care needs

The process of finding out people's care needs is called *assessment*. The obvious starting place is to find out what the person can do for themselves, how they cope in different situations, and what help is already available to them.

You should already know something about assessments; when you applied for this GNVQ course, you will have gone through an assessment yourself. People wanting help from caring agencies have to go through a very similar process.

Activity 1

• Can you describe the assessment process for selecting people to come on to the course?

• Did you know it was going on?

• Who did the assessing?

• What did you have to do?

Discuss this in small groups for about ten minutes with the other people on the course. Write out a list of the things you had to do in order to secure your place on the course.

The process you are likely to have gone through, was filling in a written application form, having an interview, and references being requested from your last school, college or employer.

CARE ASSESSMENT

There are different methods of obtaining a care assessment (this is also covered in Chapter 3, see pages 94–95). This may be through:

1 *professional referral*, most commonly the family doctor
2 *self-referral*, either in person, in writing, or by phone
3 *referral by others*, usually a relative or informal carer.
4 *referral by emergency services*, which can actually be covered by one of the three above, depending upon the circumstances at the time of the referral.

If it is decided from this first contact that this person has been referred to the right place, the first part of the assessment is to decide whether they need care services. This is often called a *'simple assessment'*. Once this has been determined, they will then be seen by the person or persons who will make the full (or 'complex') assessment: the *assessor* or *assessors*.

The assessor may be a doctor if the person in need goes to a doctor's surgery; a nurse if they go to a casualty department, or a social worker if they are in touch with a social services office. They may then be referred for a more specialist assessment service, provided for example by community occupational therapists, paediatricians, geriatricians, psychiatrists or psychologists. Sometimes a multi-disciplinary team will undertake the assessment, especially when the needs are quite complicated.

ASSESSMENT METHODS

Although there are some very specialist assessment methods such as X-rays and laboratory testing, most carers are involved in more general methods. These are the same as the procedures you went through to get a place at college: *interview, observation*, and *reports.*

Interview

This is usually when one person talks to another to find out about them, and what it is they want or need. It is sometimes a panel of people who speak to the individual. Occasionally it is not an individual who is interviewed, but a group such as a family, or a few people who are seen to have the same general needs, or who are in the same situation (people who all suffer the same disease or disability).

What you should remember in caring is that not everybody is able to communicate in the same way in an interview situation.

Activity 2

 Write down what would be different, if anything, about interviews for the following groups of people:
* deaf people
* blind people
* people with learning difficulties
* people with speech impairment
* people whose first language is not English
* young children (say what age group you have chosen)

Now that you have identified the specific arrangements which you feel are necessary, how do you think they could be overcome?

Divide into groups, and discuss one situation

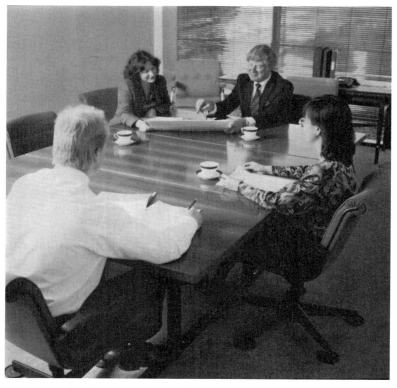

Figure 6.1   *Sometimes a multi-disciplinary team will undertake assessment, especially when the client's needs are*
complicated

each, and then organise a role-play to show the other groups how you think the interview could take place.

Who would be involved? Obviously the client and the assessor or assessors, but who else do you think could or should be there? Think about other members of the family, translators, advocates, legal advisors, union representatives, and representatives from charities (e.g. Spina Bifida Society, SCOPE, MIND, etc.). If you do not know what some of these words mean, or need to find out more about specific voluntary organisations, use the library to do some research. Also, see Chapter 3, pages 83–94.

Interviews do not always take place in an office. They can be in the client's own home, in a car, or even in the park. There may be situations involving homeless people, or those who do not want other members of their family to know what is going on.

The interview should give you a lot of background information to the current needs, but the next phase of assessment is also a very important one, especially when there are verbal communication difficulties.

Observation

This is something that takes place during interviews as well as away from interview situations. Assessments do not always have a formal interview as a part of the process, but will always have an element of observation.

Observation is watching someone. You do it all the time, but you may not be conscious of it. Do you usually know when your friends are in a bad mood, or a good mood, or excited about something? And the moods of your relatives, teachers, lecturers, workmates? People who go into caring are usually quite sensitive to emotions, but it is sometimes easier to tell by observing someone what sort of a mood they are in when you have known the person for a little while. With a stranger, it is easy to be mistaken in your assessment by making judgements on a small amount of information.

The most obvious things that are observed are physical condition and behaviour. By physical condition, we do not mean a medical diagnosis: we mean looking at a person and seeing if they are small or large, a child or an adult, male or female, and some racial characteristics, e.g. is the skin white, black, or yellow? If it is yellow, is this racial or an illness in a white person? This is an instance where other factors have to be taken into account before conclusions are reached.

Physical disability may also be obvious to an observer, such as whether the person has two legs and two arms and if they seem to be functioning properly, whether they are blind, and use aids such as a wheelchair, spectacles or a hearing aid. Chapter 4 covers all the main points on communication and observation skills which you need for this section.

Reports

Gathering information from other people is another important aspect of the assessment process. Even when people are talking about the same thing, they often see it in different ways. The importance of this method increases greatly when the client is unable to communicate with you directly. The obvious main sources of this sort of information are relatives, friends and any other care workers who may be involved already. They can tell you what has been happening and what the needs of the client are from their point of view.

CASE STUDY 1

'Mrs T' appears to be an elderly lady. She is small and has a forward stoop; she has grey hair, and many wrinkles on her face. Her skin is very tight, and the shape of the bones show through. Her clothes are good quality, and quite clean apart from food stains around the front.

She speaks with an educated accent, and says her name is Sally Smith. The police have brought Mrs T to a casualty department. They were called by a farmer who said that she was there in the early hours of the morning asking to see her parents. She was very agitated and distressed, saying that her parents would be worried about her coming home late from school.

CASE STUDY 2

Chris is 22, and had been out horse riding when a dog startled the horse, and she was thrown to the ground. The landing had been very awkward, and resulted in a broken neck. Chris has been in hospital for many months, and is now in a specialist spinal injuries unit. A discharge home has to be planned.

CASE STUDY 3

Andrew is 44 and has bouts of depression. He is frequently in and out of hospital. He lives alone, and says he has no friends; he seems to be locked in a repetitive pattern of heavy drinking followed by suicide attempts. He is in hospital once again, and plans need to be made for his discharge home.

CASE STUDY 4

Kesi is 4 years old, and lives with his mother and two older sisters. His father works abroad, and so mother has the responsibility for day-to-day care of the family. She has many problems with Kesi, whom she describes as over-active and beyond her control. He cannot sit still for a minute, and is always getting himself into risky situations. He tries to climb from windows, walks out into the road without looking, and climbs whenever he can.

He goes to a playgroup on three mornings a week. His mother has come to the social services to ask for help.

Activity 3

 Using the case histories here, decide how you are going to get information which will help in the preparation of a care plan for each person. If you do not think there is enough information in the case study, then make some up yourself to extend the study.

Write a short report of what information you think you would get from:

- an interview with the client
- observation of the client
- reports from other people involved
- other people you would speak to

Use role-play if you wish, and video-recording if the facilities are available.

CARE SETTINGS

As you will have learned from the information in the course so far, people are looked after in a variety of settings. The setting will affect the type of care given, and the care plan drawn up.

Care settings include

- residential homes
- nursing homes
- health care services
- day care services
- domiciliary services

Residential homes

Residential homes are places where people with similar care needs live, are looked after and enabled to lead as independent and enjoyable lives as possible. Their needs are usually not of a very high level (although dependency levels are rising all the time), and concern mainly physical needs such as help with the general matters of day-to-day living. The home will provide warmth, food and laundry services, plus help with mobility if required.

Old people's homes come into this category, as do many homes for people with learning difficulties. A few establishments for people with physical disabilities are residential homes. There are also a number of residential facilities for people recovering from a mental illness.

Nursing homes

These are for those people who need a greater level of care, and some element of nursing and/or medical care. They may need specialist medication administered, dressings changed, or be unable to move without help.

Nursing homes must have qualified nurses on duty at all times; this is not required in residential homes.

Health care services

These services are mainly centred on hospitals (both NHS and private), although more are moving out to health centres in some places. Practice nurses, and GP's are giving treatment in health centres which would once have been referred to hospitals.

Day care services

Day care services are now found throughout health and social care provision. To some degree, schools can be classed as a day care service. All the other forms of child care can be included in this category; day nurseries, creche, play groups, child minders and so on.

Many hospitals provide day facilities for minor surgery, where the patient arrives in the morning, has their operation and goes home when the effects have worn off in the evening.

Other day care services are for five (or sometimes seven) days a week and are pro-

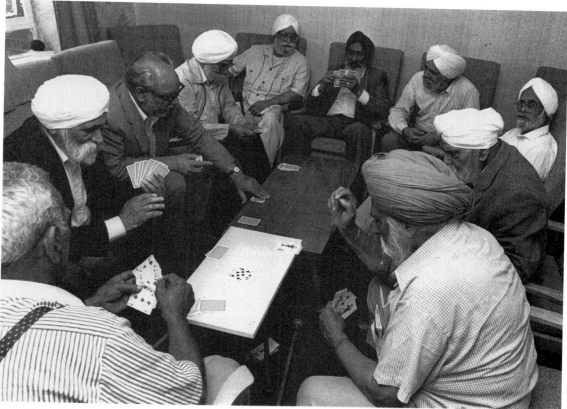

Figure 6.2   *Day centres which bring together people who share a common culture and interests are especially successful*

vided for specific client groups such as people with learning difficulties, elderly people, people with physical disabilities, and people recovering from mental illness.

Domiciliary services

The major care setting, of course, is the client's own home. Informal carers are the main group of people who look after others. They may need help from the statutory and voluntary carers, and people from these groups provide a domiciliary service, i.e. visiting people in their own homes and providing the required service, as dictated by the care plan.

CARE PLANS

The next task, and in the opinion of many of the assessors involved the most difficult one, is that of putting the care plan together. This is a statutory responsibility for social services departments in England and Wales, and health and social services boards in Northern Ireland.

A care plan should be created by using the information gained during an interview and what was noted from observation and third party reports.

There are set phases within a care plan:

1 The *Assessment* process (discussed above)
2 *Goal Setting:* this is deciding on the prior-

ity of the needs, and how best to meet those needs.

3 *Implementation*, or putting the service into operation to meet the identified need.

4 When the care plan has been implemented there has to be regular *monitoring* to check that it is working, and doing what it is supposed to be doing.

5 At set points (such as each week, each month, or even once a year depending upon the situation) there will be a formal *Review* and *Evaluation* to see if any major changes are required.

Examples of care plans

Mrs T

For Mrs T, the first thing may be a physical examination by the doctor in casualty, while the police try to find out who she really is, and where she has come from.

The first goal will be to rule out any physical illness. There are a number of possible reasons why people may become confused and wander off; some of these reasons are physical and some are psychological. If an illness is diagnosed, it may be that the care plan is to admit her to hospital and give her the necessary treatment. If no illness is found, then the goal may be to return her home and assess again for what support will be needed there.

This can only be done if the second goal is met, and that is to find out who she is and where she is missing from. The goals which follow will be different if she is found to be living alone, living with relatives, or missing from an old people's home. Each situation will require a different care plan to be developed, and Mrs T will have to be involved as much as possible in deciding what these goals are. If she is unable to take a full part in this process, then somebody else could be involved on her behalf; relatives or an advocate from a voluntary organisation, for instance.

Chris

For Chris, the goals will be more long term, as a full assessment of capabilities will have been undertaken in the hospital and the spinal injuries unit. Physical ability will be a deciding factor in what care is needed, and the amount of independence possible after returning home. A major goal to discuss is where home is to be.

Monitoring will be on an ongoing basis, and review and evaluation may initially need to be fairly frequent, but as the situation settles down, could eventually be done only twice a year.

Chris can be very closely involved in the whole process. The damage done was physical, and thinking and communication are no problem at all.

Andrew

Andrew can be involved in agreeing and setting goals, particularly at points between bouts of depression. He does have some insight, and knows what is happening. This does not stop him acting self-destructively when he is affected by depression, but afterwards he does recognise that he needs help. When he is suffering from depression, he may need somebody to speak on his behalf.

The goals could be to encourage him to go into situations where he meets other people and develops interests, which will stop him spending so much time thinking about himself.

Kesi

Kesi himself is unlikely to agree that he needs help, or that there is any problem at all. His mother certainly wants help, and his sisters may do as well. The initial goal could be to have a specialist assessment to try and find out why he is so over-active. This can be a psychological assessment as well as a physical assessment (there are some allergies which can cause this type of behaviour, as well as complicated emotional reasons).

CLIENT
PARTICIPATION

As we have mentioned, it is important to involve the person who will be receiving the care as much as possible. All matters should be discussed with them in the most appropriate way. 'Appropriate ways' may be a little more time consuming than straightforward conversation, but there are ways to do this as you should have found out from your earlier role-plays.

You also have to bear in mind the practicality of involving clients in care plans; how realistic is it to ask a baby how they feel about having a vaccination? Or a toddler about going to a playgroup?

It is a different matter where a person can understand but not respond verbally. For example, planning rehabilitation after a stroke which has affected speech; people who are deaf with no speech; and some people with severe learning difficulties who have never learned to speak. However they should always be involved, and you may need to help them communicate.

Methods

There are different ways of involving clients in matters which concern them. The first is allowing them some freedom of choice in their day-to-day affairs. You have to decide what you are going to wear at the start of each day, and it has to be appropriate for what you are going to do. The same applies to clients being cared for. The difference is

that they may need some help to choose, and this includes guidance. Would mothers let their children out in the snow wearing only summer clothes? Is it sensible to let an old lady like Mrs T go out in the rain in her dressing gown?

Carers have to show respect, and support their clients, but they also have to promote health and well-being, which includes self esteem and self image.

Allowing people to choose when and how they wish to have a bath and shower is an example of common courtesy. If someone is reluctant ever to bath or shower, all your best interpersonal skills will be needed. Confrontation is not the answer; warmth, humour and gentle persuasion can be very effective.

Other matters which can be negotiated and agreed upon with clients are, for example, the time that help arrives to get people out of bed or to put them to bed. This is not only in a residential setting, but in the community home care services. This choice should be easier in a residential setting than in the community, where a list of people have to be visited in an area within given times by the home care staff who may only work from 8 pm to 11 pm.

What food people are offered is another area where choice can be given, and to some degree what time it is eaten; but it is difficult to cope in a residential establishment such as an old people's home when the cook is there only for certain times, and everybody wants to eat something different at a different time.

The important point to bear in mind is that choice is a matter of *consultation* and *consent*, and not an open book of everyone getting what they want, when they want it, all the time. Life is just not like that, is it?

It is essential that while reading this section, you take into account all the information covered in Chapter 4.

ADVOCATES

Where clients are unable to speak up for themselves they may wish to appoint an advocate: a person who speaks on behalf of another. This may be, as we have discussed, because that person has some sort of physical or learning disability, and cannot speak directly for themselves. It may be purely nervousness, and fear of speaking out, especially if it is in some sort of public place, or to a few people at the same time.

You may have done some advocacy yourself, and not realised it. Have you ever been in the situation at school where a friend is very upset, and sobbing so much that they have trouble telling you what is the matter? A teacher then comes along and asks what is going on, and it is you that says 'Jackie has been knocked off her bike by some boys in the schoolyard', or 'Julie has fallen out with her parents/boyfriend/sister', etc. If Jackie or Julie want to go home, or to sit somewhere quietly, and you ask the teacher if they can do that, you are acting as an *advocate* on behalf of that other person.

The most well known type of advocate is the lawyer, who will speak in court on behalf of people on trial. The lawyer will find out what his or her client wants to say, and that will be what he or she says in court. Another example may be the union representative in industrial tribunals. They could be speaking up for someone who feels that they have been unfairly dismissed, for example.

An advocate does not have to be an official, however, they can be a relative or friend who has been nominated by the client. All they have to do is advocate the client's views to the care assessor. This may be that they want only vegetarian meals, no male carers, no visits after 7 pm, respite care only at Stoughton Hall, etc.

If somebody wishes to speak up on their

OAKWOOD ADVOCACY SERVICE
2 Advocacy workers required

Sinclair & Sons is a solicitor's firm specialising in mental health and disability law. The firm has contracted to provide an advocacy service for mental health service users in the Oakwood Health District. This venture is funded and strongly supported by Oakwood Health Commissioning Agency. The project is initially funded for three years.

We are seeking 2 advocacy workers to work in hospitals and the community for 28 hours per week each. Candidates should have:

  a commitment to representing the interests of mental health service users;

  a knowledge of mental health services;

  experience and/or knowledge of advocacy;

  an ability to work effectively with mental health service providers in pursuit of the user's expressed wishes;

  word processing skills.

We are an equal opportunities employer.

For further information contact:

Oakwood Advocacy Service
Sinclair & Sons
Signet House, 49 Barrett Road
London EC2M 4AH

Figure 6.3   *An advocacy service*

---

own behalf, this is known as *self-advocacy*. Help may be needed in enabling clients to do this. It may be something they have never done before, and are very shy about.

- How did you feel giving your first presentation to the class?
- Preparing what you are going to say in advance is a great help, and writing it down so that you can look at it, read it, and change it about.
- Practising how you are going to say it is another way to prepare. Stand in front of a mirror and say what you think you will need to say.

- Clients may need to be given self-confidence by being told that they are able to do it, and that it is alright to read out something they have written beforehand.
- Sometimes a role-play, the same as you do on your GNVQ course sometimes, will help prepare clients for self-advocacy.
- If it is possible, you could introduce them to the people who will be in the meeting before it happens, so that some faces are familiar.

Scenario

Luke is a teenager being looked after by a local authority. Every six months, Luke's situation has to be reviewed. The people involved will include the social workers and teachers who see him regularly, parents and/or foster parents, other care staff, plus one or two other people who may not know Luke personally at all.

One of the things that is likely to happen is that Luke will be asked how he is getting on, and what he would like to happen over the next six months. It is obviously much better if Luke is confident enough to say himself what he wants, although he does have the option of an advocate.

Activity 4

Organise a role-play of Luke's review meeting.

You could start by helping Luke to prepare for what he is going to say, or you could leave him to go into the meeting unprepared and shrug his shoulders when asked questions.

There could be two variations on the theme; one with an advocate speaking on behalf of Luke, the other with Luke speaking for himself.

1 The situation may be that Luke is living away from home and wants to return. He is in care because of offences he has committed, such as stealing from cars and shops. One of the questions asked would be how he intends to stay out of trouble, and what he is going to do to stop himself becoming bored, or mixing with the people who got him into trouble before.

2 Another situation may be that Luke is in a residential school because he was always playing truant from school when he lived at home. His parents want him back, and Luke would be asked about going to school if he lived back at home, and what his future plans might be.

3 You can make up your own story about Luke, and role play whatever fits in with that.

Decide who is going to be at the meeting, and at what point you are going to start the role-play. This could be before the meeting, with Luke telling an advocate what he wants to say (the advocate is not there to give advice, only to say what Luke wants to be said), or it could be with the care worker helping Luke prepare himself for what he wants to say in the meeting.

All of this could be video-taped, and also used as discussion/evidence for the Communication and Interpersonal Relationships unit (Unit 4).

APPEALS AND COMPLAINTS PROCEDURES

When a care plan has been designed, the person who is to receive it, or their representative, may not be happy with it, or certain parts of it. If this is the case, the social services must have a *complaints* procedure in place, and an *appeals* procedure. The appeals route is only used after the complaints procedure has been used, but has failed to solve the points of disagreement.

A complaint may also arise, for example,

when the early morning call comes too late or too early, or meals on wheels arrives cold, or the laundry service leaves sheets and towels grubby. This should be dealt with by the care manager, and lead to the problem being resolved.

An appeal may occur when the care plan states that two hours a week of home care assistance will be provided, and the client thinks that two hours a day would be more appropriate. Or that respite care is allowed once a year when the client wants it to be four times a year.

There should be set procedures available from your local social services department or health and social services board; ask your school or college library if they have copies for you to look at.

CLIENT INVOLVEMENT IN SHAPING THE CARE ENVIRONMENT

Client groups

Sometimes there may be an issue in a sheltered housing scheme, day centre or residential centre which affects all or most of the people who live there. When an individual makes their views known, it may not have very much effect. If a few people can get together and make the same point, it is more likely that notice will be taken.

When this strategy is made more formal, the people who have joined together become the 'residents' committee', 'users' group', or 'day care members' group', or something similar. They can then be approached to take part in setting out the rules and regulations for everybody involved in that facility.

Residents' committees or user groups can be asked to put together a report for the management of the scheme or the day centre (which could be in the statutory, voluntary or private sectors of care provision). They can also be asked to send representatives to management meetings to state the point of view of the users.

CASE STUDY 5

Stoughton Hall is a private residential home with twelve bungalows in the grounds. Elderly people move into the bungalows when they are still able to look after themselves, but want the security of knowing that help is readily available should they need it.

The people in the bungalows see themselves as different from those living in the main building, and feel that they should have more freedom of choice. One of their main complaints is that they are not allowed to keep pets other than cage birds or fish. The residents' committee is made up of people from the bungalows and from the main building. The bungalow people want their own group to put forward their point of view.

They elect to send a representative to the management committee to put forward this idea. When this is agreed to, they will move on to their next goal of allowing bungalow residents to keep cats or dogs if they want to. They consider pets to be very therapeutic, and an essential part of their care plans.

In order to achieve this aim, they will be acting as a pressure group.

Activity 5

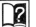

- Look at Case Studies 1–6.
- Design a leaflet which will tell the families involved in Cases 1–4, or new people becoming involved in 5 or 6, how their care needs will be assessed, and how they will be involved.
- For either 5 or 6, design a poster which will be put up in the entrance area so that the information is easily seen and understood by anyone visiting.

CASE STUDY 6

The mental health day centre has a members' group, and elections are held every six months. People who go to the day centre tend to stay for a long time. There is a policy of having as few rules and regulations as possible, and allowing people the freedom to come and go as they wish. This also includes only taking part in what they want to.

A problem has arisen with a small number of people coming in only at lunch time, eating their very cheap meal, and then leaving. The majority of members are not happy with this, as the daily meal is a group exercise, with the meal being planned in the morning. Some members then have to go shopping, some make the meal, and others lay the tables and then clear and do the washing up. The people who just come in and eat are taking no part in any of this. The members' group want to change the rules to make them have to do a job as well as eat.

Participation in such tasks as going shopping, cooking, and cleaning up are a part of individual care plans as well as the group care plan. Some people with mental health problems find such simple things as discussing with other people, reaching decisions, and going into a shop very difficult to do, and need a great deal of help and encouragement. The daily meal helps many people to do these things with support.

THE NHS AND COMMUNITY CARE ACT 1990

This will have been mentioned many times during your GNVQ course; it is the main piece of legislation covering the care of all adult client groups, and some children.

One of the things a local authority has to do as a part of this Act is to provide a community care plan for their area every year. This is to tell people what services will be provided, and how much money is available for them. What services are provided is something which has to be discussed widely with all the interested parties, but it would be an impossible task to speak to every individual concerned. Letters or questionnaires are sent to User Groups and Residents' Committees, and it is up to them to consult individuals and send back a consensus view. Also involved are national voluntary organisations such as SCOPE, MIND, MENCAP, Help the Aged, (usually through their local offices), and local voluntary groups which only operate in that local authority area (see Chapter 3, page 86 for further information).

The legislation says that

it will be the responsibility of the social services authority to design care arrangements in line with individual needs, in consultation with the client and other care professionals, and within available resources.

Consultation with community groups, some of which will be 'pressure groups' set up to achieve a specific aim, must take place on the overall design of services.

The day-to-day delivery of these services is a matter for the social services departments or health and social services boards to decide, but individual clients should be involved where it is a component of their personal care plan.

The phrase 'within available resources' is causing some problems. Social services are running out of money, and having to keep a close eye on how much care plans are costing. Some people are not getting the service they think they should have, or having services reduced. The clients involved are going to appeal, and some cases have been to court for decisions to be made. The courts have agreed that the social services have only a set amount of money, and must keep within those spending limits.

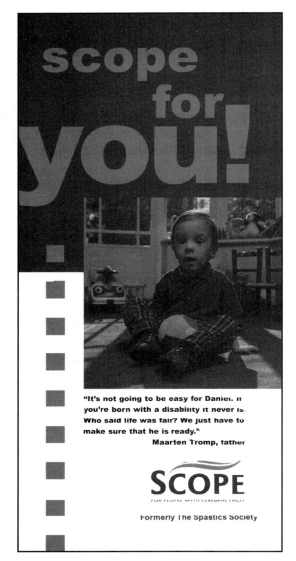

Figure 6.4 *SCOPE is a voluntary organisation for people with cerebral palsy*

Allocation of funds to purchase care

There is some discussion about letting clients have a sum of money, and organising their own packages of care. The government has not agreed to allow this to happen yet. They may be worried that the money will not be used as it was supposed to be; i.e. people will use it to go on holiday, or for something other than care needs. Permission may be given at some time though, and you can find out by keeping an eye on weekly magazines such as *Community Care* and *Caring Times*.

The Community Care Plan produced every year is one way that clients can influence the allocation of funds; individuals are allowed to send in their views, but obviously a group view such as from a pressure group representing hundreds or thousands of clients is likely to have more influence. Many voluntary organisations fulfil this role of pressure group and representing client views, and say where they think money should be spent the following year.

- Mental health groups such as MIND or SANE may say that more money should be given to help people recovering from a mental illness; RADAR may say that more should go to help disabled people, and so on.

- The User Groups described in Case Studies 5 and 6 may also be involved in the allocation of funds on a smaller scale. The management may have a sum of money to spend, e.g. on decorating rooms within Stoughton Hall. They may ask the client representatives to decide on which rooms should be done. The other rooms will have to wait until more money is available.

- The day centre group may have to decide whether to purchase a mini-bus or pay for a week's holiday for the members. Playgroups may have to decide whether to buy play equipment or modernise the toilet area.

Activity 6

 Organise a role-play of the above situations. Play the part of the management committees of
- Stoughton Hall
- The day centre
- A playgroup

and decide how a donation of £1000 will be spent.

In Stoughton Hall, you will have to decide which rooms should be decorated: the communal rooms (dining room, lounge, library, conservatory), the bedrooms, bathrooms, toilets, kitchen, or the offices.

If you choose the bedrooms, which ones? There is not enough money to do all of them.

Will it be the ones of the people who have lived there the longest? The empty rooms which can be done more easily? The rooms which were decorated the longest time ago?

Whatever you decide to do, give the reasons for your choice. There is no 'right answer'.

Individual needs

At the end of this section, you should have:

- Summarised the needs of individuals in care settings
- Identified and given examples of health and social care settings in the community
- Described how individuals care needs are met in different care settings
- Described the roles of care workers in meeting individual needs

HEALTH AND SOCIAL CARE SETTINGS

Health and social care settings are the places where people are cared for. These are covered in some detail in Mandatory Unit 3. If you have not done this yet, turn to Chapter 3 and use the material from sections one and two for your portfolio. Settings cover such places as hospitals, nursing homes, residential homes, day care services and domiciliary services and health care services for all client groups.

If you do not feel you have enough portfolio evidence from Unit 3, or want to cover this unit first, then this exercise will help.

Activity 7

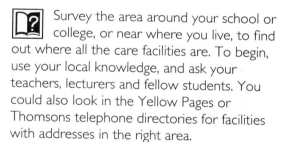 Survey the area around your school or college, or near where you live, to find out where all the care facilities are. To begin, use your local knowledge, and ask your teachers, lecturers and fellow students. You could also look in the Yellow Pages or Thomsons telephone directories for facilities with addresses in the right area.

Social services offices and health trusts may also be useful sources of information.

Remember to include facilities for all the client groups in the range:
- *Children:* nurseries, playgroups, mother and toddler groups, schools, hospitals, and anything else you think is relevant.
- *Elders:* Residential homes, day centres, luncheon clubs, Nursing homes and hospitals.
- *People with learning disabilities:* schools, hostels, day centres, specialist hospitals, group living schemes.

• *People with mental health problems:* day centres, hospitals, hostels, group living schemes, support networks.

If there are not facilities of a particular kind, or for a particular client group in the area you have chosen to look at, then find out where the nearest resource is to be found. Get to know as much as you can about it, and write a short report for your portfolio on each facility outside your area.

NEEDS OF INDIVIDUALS

The basic needs of individuals are the same, whether in care settings or not. The difference may be that when people are in care settings, they may need help to meet those needs as they are unable to do so themselves.

These are covered in other units of your GNVQ course, but to summarise, our needs can be broken down into four main groupings:

• Physical
• Intellectual
• Emotional
• Social

These can be easily remembered by thinking of *PIES*, as in apple pies or meat pies.

Physical needs include food, drink, air, warmth, exercise and freedom from pain and discomfort.

Intellectual needs are those which keep the mind active, such as reading, watching TV, going to the theatre, playing games or doing puzzles e.g. crosswords, solitaire. This can be alone or with other people, but when it is with other people, we are also meeting our social needs, and possibly emotional needs

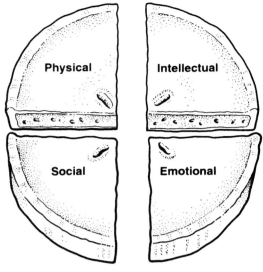

Figure 6.5   *PIES*

too, so care has to be taken when you are putting things into categories.

Emotional needs are met by having a sense of belonging; being part of a group such as a family, having confidence in yourself as a person, and knowing that you are valued by others.

Social needs include having time to relax, enjoying friendships, and taking part in things which interest us.

It is difficult to separate out these needs in reality, as they are so closely interlinked. Many needs which you can think of will go under more than one heading.

Activity 8

Draw four columns on a piece of paper, then put headings for each one of P I E and S. Read Case Studies 7 and 8, and put in each column which needs are being met by what Lucy and Walter do and what happens to them.

Some things will appear in more than one column, but this does not matter; i.e.

Physical	Intellectual	Emotional	Social
ice cream	radio	family	club

CASE STUDY 7

Lucy is twenty-two years old. She has her own room in a hostel with nine other young people. She loves music and dancing, and also painting. When she is in her room she listens to the radio, and likes the stories and plays which are on Radio 4.

She likes to play all the games she can join in, such as rounders and basketball, skipping, and anything else that is going on. She also enjoys swimming and going for walks in the country. Once a week she goes to a Gateway Club, where she can do a lot of dancing, and join in some games. On Sundays she goes out with her mother, who is nearly 70, and widowed. Occasionally she sees her older brother, who is married and has two young children. Lucy enjoys seeing them.

Her favourite food is ice cream, and she would have this for every meal if she were allowed. Lucy also has Downs' Syndrome, and often gets chest infections which need treating with antibiotics. The hostel staff make sure she takes her medicines when the doctor prescribes them.

CASE STUDY 8

Walter lives alone in a small bungalow. He watches television, listens to local radio, and reads cowboy novels. He has a dog, and enjoys taking it for walks two or three times a day. When he is out with the dog he often meets people and has a chat.

On weekend evenings, he likes to go to the pub for an hour before bedtime. He does not drink much, but enjoys the company.

He gets the Daily Mirror delivered every morning, reads this over breakfast, and usually does the crossword after taking the dog for a walk.

Walter will be 76 this year, has diabetes and only one leg as a result of a war wound. His sight is failing, and he needs a magnifying glass to read his paper. The novels are large print versions from the local library.

The district nurse calls on him each day to change a dressing on his stump, and see that his blood sugar is alright.

Physical needs

Physical needs include a *healthy diet*; this is covered in Chapter 1. Turn to pages 7–10 to cover the material for this, or use the evidence from this already in your portfolio.

The physical needs of some individuals are met by the provision of specialist equipment. Some of these items you will see every day, and may even use yourself. Look around you and see how many people are wearing spectacles. Some may have false teeth, (which are not so easy to see), or hearing aids.

Many people you see out and about use walking aids, the most common being a walking stick. Others are walking frames (e.g. Zimmer frames) or trolleys. A few people may be on crutches, and others in wheelchairs.

Activity 9

 Go to the nearest town, shopping centre or market in small groups. Spend 20 minutes or so in one spot looking at the people passing you by.

- Make a note of how many people make use of some sort of aid to help with daily living.
- Remember children in pushchairs, as well as the other things mentioned above.
- When looking at walking sticks, how many of them are white ones, and what does this signify?
- What would a person carry a red and white walking stick for?
- How many cars have an orange badge on them? What does this mean?

The things you have seen around you are all examples of how some people's care needs are met when they are out and about in the community. At home, some people have aids and adaptations in their houses to help them. Some adaptations are quite simple, and help everybody living in that house or flat: e.g. fit-

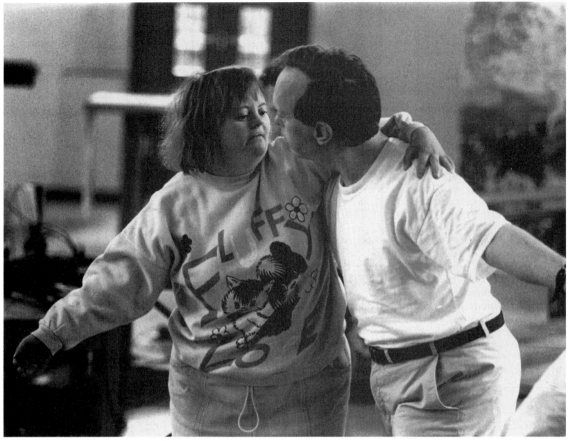

Figure 6.6   *Social events such as dances can help people make friends*

ting a downstairs and upstairs toilet, a shower as well as a bath. Other adaptations may be much more specific, such as lifts or stairlifts, ramps and grab-handles at points around the house or flat.

There are many other smaller aids and adaptations available, from adapted knives and forks to low level cookers and sliding sinks. You can find out more about these by getting a catalogue from Boots, or from another retail outlet listed in the Thomson Directory under 'Disabled Equipment'. You could also write to organisations such as:

Disabled Living Foundation
380–384 Harrow Rd
London W9 2HU

Remember to include a stamped addressed envelope for the reply. You could also visit a display centre within reach of your school or college.

Nursing care and medical care

This is something most of us will need at some point during our lives. It may be just a visit to the doctor, or an immunisation from the school nurse, but we probably all have some contact with doctors and nurses at some time. Some people need a lot more of this type of care than others, usually only for specified periods of their lives.

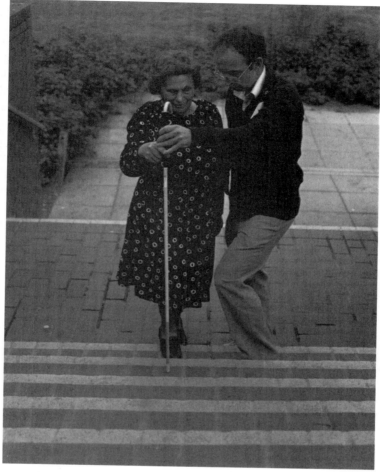

Figure 6.7   *Someone who has lost their sight will need to learn new ways of getting around safely*

CASE STUDY 9

Hilda lives with her cat in an upstairs maisonette on a warden-controlled site. She is a plump, friendly lady who likes nothing better than a chat over a cup of tea with anybody who visits her. She knows everything that is going on in the neighbourhood, despite not being able to get out much.

The reason for this is her arthritis. It is affecting all her joints, and she is having increasing difficulty not just with walking, but with gripping anything. This means that she has trouble with washing and dressing, going to the toilet, and preparing meals and drinks. Turning on taps, opening bottles, and getting a grip of small controls on the cooker are really difficult for her.

CASE STUDY 10

Colin has a ground floor flat waiting for him to move into. He is 23, has lots of friends, and used to enjoy racing around on his motorbike when he wasn't working in his father's garage. That was before his accident. He was alone, it was late at night, and nobody saw what happened. He was found in the road with a broken back in the early hours of the morning.

After going to the local hospital, he was transferred to a spinal injuries unit. He has been there for about 18 months now, and is ready to move out to his flat. He has learned to use a wheelchair, but has no feeling or movement below his waist. Weight training has made his upper body very strong, and he is taking part in sports competitions. He wishes to be as independent as possible.

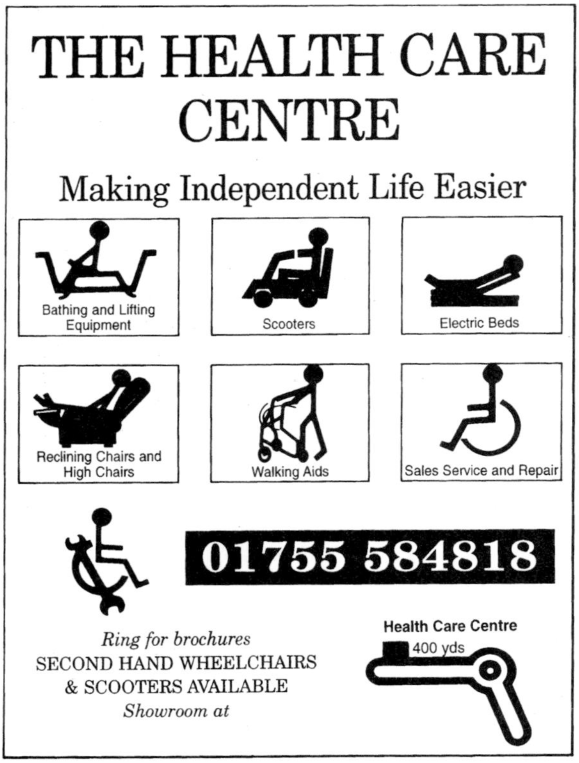

THE HEALTH CARE CENTRE

Making Independent Life Easier

Bathing and Lifting Equipment

Scooters

Electric Beds

Reclining Chairs and High Chairs

Walking Aids

Sales Service and Repair

01755 584818

Ring for brochures
SECOND HAND WHEELCHAIRS
& SCOOTERS AVAILABLE
Showroom at

Health Care Centre
400 yds

Figure 6.8   *There are many local centres selling aids and equipment for disabled and elderly people*

Activity 10

Using the catalogues you have obtained, decide what aids and adaptations would best help the people described in Case Studies 9 and 10.

- What sort of nursing and medical care would Colin have needed from the moment he was found in the road until he moves into his flat?
- Hilda has a fall and fractures her hip. She calls the warden, who calls the GP, who arranges for her to be taken to hospital. The consultant decides that she needs a hip replacement. Find out about the nursing and medical care she will receive during this process.

Social needs

These can be met by both formal and informal methods in care settings. In residential homes or day centres, for example, clients will be talking to each other and doing things together during the normal course of the day. This is *informal socialising*. More formal ways of encouraging socialisation are events organised by the staff or the Users' Committee (or its equivalent). These may be Bingo sessions, dances, coffee mornings, jumble sales, garden parties or fêtes. Some of these will involve people with whom the residents or users are not normally in contact. There will also be trips out to the theatre or cinema, or to the seaside or zoo, etc.

It is during these events that social relationships can be formed or strengthened, and emotional needs met.

Emotional needs can also be met during more specialised and structured meetings such as therapeutic groups of people who share the same needs.

CASE STUDY 11

Ann is afraid to go out of her house alone. She lives with her husband John and two children, and keeps everything extremely neat and tidy. The shopping can only be done when John is at home, and the children go to school with friends' parents. Ann is collected and taken to the day centre by Jane, a community psychiatric nurse (CPN) on Mondays and Fridays. These are the days when there is a 'phobic group' held. All the people attending have an irrational fear of one sort or another, and agoraphobia (which Ann has) is one of the more common phobias.

The group get together and talk about their fears and how they affect their lives. They also make suggestions to each other on how to cope in different situations. There are only a maximum of ten people in the group at any one time, and between the meetings Jane sees each of them for individual counselling.

Activity 11

- Write notes about which of Ann's needs are being met, and how they are being met.

Valuing individuals

Some of this subject is covered in Chapters 2 and 4.

When you are looking after other people, it is important to show them that they are individuals, and that they matter. One way that we do this is in the way that we speak to them, and another is in the way we act toward them.

People need personal space, and standing too close can be very threatening. It also means that eye contact may be lost, and also the opportunity to observe body language. Standing too far away can also be an insult; is it because they smell? Also, if you have to speak too loudly, the conversation is no longer intimate and private. When the other person has a hearing impairment, allowances have to be made for this, perhaps by only speaking of private matters in a private situation, such as their own bedroom or in an office.

One of the first things to find out about people in your care is how they like to be addressed. Does John Thompson like to be called John, Johnny, Mr Thompson, or even Tommy? Perhaps Grandad, Pops, or Chuck are preferable to him – but not unless he says so.

The best way to find out is to consult, i.e. ask him. The same goes for many other everyday things such as does he want tea or coffee; Cornflakes or rice krispies, brown bread or white? Involving clients in decision making should be done as a matter of course to the best of their ability. Ask their opinions, put to them the available options, dis-

cuss the pros and cons of each possible choice.

CASE STUDY 12

John Thompson is an elderly man who lives alone. He is finding it harder to cope with looking after himself as he gets older, but does not want to leave his own home. A day attendance place is arranged for him at a residential home on Mondays, Wednesdays and Fridays from 10 am to 4 pm. He is collected and taken home by taxi. He has a bad heart and is on a low salt diet, and likes to eat small amounts of food every couple of hours. When he has been attending for a week or two, his social worker suggests he might like to move into the home rather than coming for three days a week.

Activity 12

- Write down the things that the care workers at the home would need to find out about him so that they can look after him properly.
- Role-play a conversation between the social worker and Mr Thompson to discuss the possibility of him moving into the residential home, bearing in mind the need for consultation and participation in decision making (as well as all the material from Chapter 4 on Interpersonal skills).

Intellectual needs

Children's intellectual needs are met by going to school until they are 16 years old; some then go on to college and higher education. Other client groups have their intellectual needs met in less formal ways such as watching television, listening to the radio, reading newspapers, magazines and books or taking part in other pastimes which require some thought and give mental stimulation.

Adults of all ages often continue to learn by going on day release courses, night school, or signing on for distance learning such as the Open University.

We have discussed earlier some of the ways that clients in residential care can meet their intellectual needs, and they can also do all the things mentioned here.

Care workers

Information on this is a part of your work for Chapter 3. The notes here should act as a reminder, but you can use your work from the third section of that chapter as evidence here as well.

Care assistants/Nursing assistants

These are the people who do the majority of the hands-on care in residential homes and sometimes in day centres. Those who work in hospitals are called health care assistants, or nursing assistants and those who visit people to care for them in their own homes are known as domiciliary care assistants, (also domiciliary support workers, home care assistants and home helps – and sometimes community care workers or health support workers). As a result of the NHS and Community Care Act 1990, jobs are changing and so are the job-titles.

The work they do is centred on the physical needs of people: making sure that they are warm, clean and fed. They should be doing this in a way which respects individuality and choice.

They will also be involved in meeting the social, emotional and intellectual needs of their clients, but this is unlikely to be included in their job descriptions. Clients and patients have more daily contact with care assistants and nursing assistants than any other group of care workers, and tend to have a much closer relationship with them than the doctor or district nurse, who visit less frequently.

The private and voluntary sectors are creating more of these jobs; look in your local papers and see if you can find adverts like this one:

Qualified Nurses & Experienced Carers

Urgently required by
Associated Social Care
for a variety of work in this area.
We can offer excellent rates of pay and flexible hours.

Please call 01234 500000

Figure 6.9 *A care assistant job advert*

Social workers

The name 'social worker' is a general term, and people with this job title work in a wide variety of settings. Most are employed by local authority social services departments (or health and social services boards in Northern Ireland). They tend to work in specialist teams, and so will specialise in working with certain client groups.

They are generally known as 'field' social workers; i.e. they go out to visit people in their homes. There are teams which specialise in working with:

- elderly people
- disabled people
- children and families
- child abuse
- learning difficulties
- juvenile justice problems

The basic qualification is the same; it is the personal choice of job which differs.

Although most work in local authorities, there are social workers who are employed by voluntary organisations such as the NSPCC, ASBAH (the Association for Spina Bifida and Hydrocephalus), the Family Welfare Association, Childrens' Society, Barnardo's, and others. A few are employed by solicitors, and others are in private practice. Some are employed by big organisations such as WH Smith, Boots, SSAFA (The Soldiers, Sailors And Air Force Association) and the National Union of Mineworkers.

Their primary task is one of assessment, and then of finding the right answer to the assessed needs. This may be provided by the social workers themselves in the form of counselling or giving advice, or arranged from any part of the mixed economy of care.

Residential Social Workers (RSWs)

Some social workers work in places where their clients live, such as children's homes, or hostels for recovering mentally ill, or for people with learning difficulties. They may then be known as residential social workers. They do not necessarily have the same qualifications as field social workers, and so many people start their careers as RSWs, and become field workers after they have experience and training.

Physiotherapists

Their job is to help people maintain as much bodily movement as possible. They do this through the use of exercise and manipulation, and the application of heat and electricity where necessary. Most work within the NHS, but there are a growing number who are self-employed, or working for private organisations such as BUPA (The British United Provident Association).

Occupational therapists

OTs assess an individual's practical abilities for day-to-day living, and sometimes for the job that an individual does or may want to do. They will then advise on techniques or aids and adaptations which will help that person. So they may re-design a house to take account of a newly acquired disability, or provide bath seats and long-handled taps for somebody becoming arthritic and losing their ability to grip objects.

Psychologists

These are people who study mental processes, development and behaviour. In the context of caring, they often make assessments of the intellectual capabilities of people. They make recommendations on how intellectual and educational needs can be met, as in the 'statementing' process for children with special needs. They could also be involved in devising a treatment programme for Ann in Case Study 11. A psychologist might also be asked to assess Lucy's intellectual capabilities, in Case Study 7.

Counsellors

Anybody can call themselves a counsellor, although there is training to become one. Unfortunately there are so many different types of training, it is difficult to pick one that is more respected than another. Possibly the best point of contact is:

British Association for Counselling (BAC)
1 Regent Place
Rugby
Warwickshire CV21 2PJ
Tel. no.: 01788 578 328

Remember your sae.

Counsellors help people come to terms with or solve their personal problems. They do this by helping them to discover for themselves the solutions or the ability to cope in a sympathetic and supportive environment.

Many caring professionals use counselling as a tool in their everyday work. There are also professional counsellors who do that work for a living. One of the best known counselling agencies is Relate (the marriage guidance council). Another which provides bereavement counselling is:

Cruse
126 Sheen Rd
Richmond
Surrey TW9 1UR
Tel. no.: 0181 332 7227

Teachers

Teaching is often classified as a caring profession, particularly for primary age children. Teachers are also involved more directly in health and social care; many work in children's services provided by social services departments and boards. They may go out to the homes of individual students and provide a teaching service there, or work in special units for those excluded from school for one reason or another.

Teachers are found in juvenile justice teams, learning difficulties services, and hospitals. They are involved with teaching adults as well as children.

Nurses

Nurses come in many different varieties. There are currently five training routes:

- Registered general nurse
- Registered mental nurse
- Registered sick children's nurse
- Registered nurse for the mentally handicapped
- Registered midwife

After obtaining one of these qualifications, there are a wide variety of titles based on different jobs. Some of them require further training, and some do not. So an occupational health nurse looks after people at work; a school nurse looks after children at school; a district nurse visits people at home; a practice nurse works in a doctor's surgery or a health centre.

Nurses also run nursing homes or old people's homes, and may be known as an officer in charge, or a matron, or a manager. In hospitals they may be called sisters, nursing officers, or unit managers. Some move on to become health visitors, and work in the community – mainly with children, sometimes with elderly people, but also on matters of health promotion.

Doctors

Like nurses, doctors come in many different guises. The basic training is the same, and then doctors choose which area they wish to work in. The type of doctor we are most likely to come into fairly regular contact with, is the GP, General Practitioner. Others are specialist doctors to whom the GP refers patients for more specific advice:

- Paediatricians work with children
- Geriatricians work with older people
- Surgeons give treatment by surgery, and physicians give other treatments
- Pathologists work in laboratories or carry out post mortem examinations
- Psychiatrists deal with mental illness, and psycho-geriatricians with mental illness in older people.

There are other types of doctor, but these are the ones you are most likely to hear about; see Chapter 3, pages 98–100.

Delivery of care in different settings

At the end of this section you should be able to:

- Identify and give examples of care values that influence the delivery of care
- Describe how environmental factors influence the delivery of care in different care settings
- Describe how the availability of human and physical resources influence the delivery of care in different care settings

Activity 13

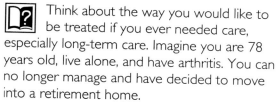 Think about the way you would like to be treated if you ever needed care, especially long-term care. Imagine you are 78 years old, live alone, and have arthritis. You can no longer manage and have decided to move into a retirement home.

- What sort of place would you like it to be?
- How would you like the staff to behave toward you?
- What would you hate most about having to rely on other people to see to all your daily needs?

CARE VALUES

In whichever setting you may be doing your caring (residential homes, nursing homes, day care, health care or domiciliary care), there are certain basic *values* which you will be expected to follow.

Values in the context of care are the *current* beliefs about:

- the right and proper way to deal with patients or clients

- the principles of valuing individuals as individuals
- preserving dignity
- encouraging independence
- allowing self-determination
- maintaining confidentiality

I say 'current' beliefs because values change. It is easy to criticise patterns of the past when care was to do things for people whether they wanted it or not, but they were the values current at that time. Large asylums, children's villages and orphanages, and the workhouses were built to care for people who had no choice in the matter.

Valuing individuals

As we have already mentioned, values today include treating each person you deal with as an individual. It is acceptable to talk about 'patients' and 'clients' (and often 'service-users' these days) collectively. But when you are working at a place regularly, it is not really acceptable to say that 'One of the patients wants to go to the toilet', or 'The fractured femur wants a bed pan'; it is far better to talk about the individual involved, so 'Mabel wants to go to the toilet', or 'Mrs Henshaw wants a bed pan'.

Whether you address them as Mabel or Mrs Henshaw is a matter of finding out about them and their likes and dislikes, and what they prefer you to call them. If you do not know a name, it is alright to ask – especially when you are on a placement from your GNVQ course and will not be expected to know everybody.

Another way of valuing individuals is by knocking at the doors of their houses, flats or rooms. Most homes for elderly people, and many nursing homes have single rooms or double rooms for their clients or patients. Many clients living at home leave doors unlocked for care workers to come and go, or give them their own keys. Even if this is the case, a knock or a shout to let them know you are there will avoid taking them by surprise.

You could find out about their food likes and dislikes to show that you value your patient's choice. Do they prefer tea or coffee; do they take sugar; brown bread or white bread, dark chocolate or milk chocolate, and so on. Think of your own likes and dislikes, and how awkward you would be to look after!

In a more general way, people can be shown respect by the way we refer to them not just individually, but collectively. It is not seen as politically correct to refer to groups such as 'the handicapped', 'the disabled', 'the elderly', or 'the mentally handicapped', for example. This seems to deny the fact that they are *people*; you could be talking about the potatoes, the luggage, or the bedding. Always refer to any group of clients as people: e.g. 'disabled people', 'people with learning difficulties', or 'elderly people'.

The ability to choose

This is sometimes referred to as just *'choice'*. We have mentioned above finding out about food likes and dislikes. The amount of choice available for this depends upon the care setting. In an individual's own home, the choice is probably limited by cost only; the client can decide what they would like, and arrange for it to be bought and prepared. In a group-living situation, such as a hospital or a retirement home, the choices will be more limited, and from a menu with a few options only. The same is true of meals on wheels; choice is limited to what is delivered.

If it were not so, the costs and the organisational structures involved would be far too high for the service to be provided at all. Imagine what it would be like if every patient in a hospital with 900 beds were to ask for a different meal to be prepared. Even 30 people on a meals on wheels round having 30 different meals would cause enormous difficulties.

MEALTIMES

It is also not always easy to allow any choice in what time food is eaten. Again, in a domiciliary situation, this may be easier than in a residential setting, but there may be organisational constraints.

In most residential settings, there will be a set time for main meals, and only a small amount of leeway possible in the time it is served. In domiciliary settings, the client may be receiving meals on wheels, or there may be a home care assistant (HCA) attending to prepare food (possibly also to feed the client). Meals on wheels will be delivered as part of a round, visiting 25–30 or more people, and individual delivery times cannot be catered for. Similarly an HCA usually has several lunchtime clients to fit in, so only a small amount of choice can be given.

PERSONAL HYGIENE

Another example of an organisational constraint is in how much choice can be given in the times of going to the toilet. Most people want to go first thing in the morning. If a client needs help, they have to wait their turn whether at home waiting for an HCA or in a residential place, where there may be a queue. They may, of course, be dependent upon the care staff to help them. If they cannot wait, this is a cause of incontinence (wetting or soiling themselves).

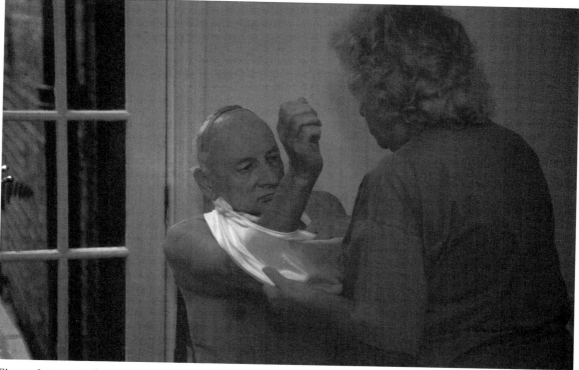

Figure 6.10   *Always ask your client what they would like to wear, and help them to do as much as possible for themselves*

CLOTHING

Clothing is another area which is sometimes a problem in residential homes. Can the residents choose what to wear, or do the care staff choose for them? Do residents have their own clothes or do they have to wear those which belong to the establishment?

Some children's homes used to have a general stock of clothes that were shared between everybody – whether they fitted properly or not!

HCAs should always ask their clients what they want to wear, not choose for them; (see Chapter 8, pages 241–42).

SELF-DETERMINATION

Self-determination is linked to these things: allowing people to determine for themselves what they would like done for them, and

how. Small matters become very important when life is reduced to the limits of a building. As we get older, our interest in outside things tends to diminish. What time you have a meal, or which day and time of day you have a bath takes on more importance than the price of clothes in the shops, and what the politicians are doing. Being able to have control over these things can enhance peace of mind and help to make life much less stressful for client and care workers alike.

DIGNITY

Dignity and privacy are other aspects of our lives which we like to see preserved. Care workers can help preserve the dignity of the people they care for by doing the things we have discussed above, e.g. using the form of address agreed by the client (Mr Smith, Mrs

Brown, Eloise, Raj, etc.). Many embarrassments can be avoided by talking quietly or in a private place, adjusting clothing which has become disarrayed, closing toilet, bathroom and bedroom doors when necessary. Dealing with incontinence or dribbling in a sensitive way can also preserve dignity. There is no need to make a fuss about it, or shout something like 'Mollie's wet herself again, come and give us a hand!'. Gently leading Mollie back to her room or the bathroom for a change of clothes, and asking a colleague quietly for help will do the job just as well, if not better.

In essence, the way you treat other people should be as close as possible to the way you would like to be treated yourself.

Activity 14

- Look at what you wrote for the activity at the beginning of this element. Can you pick out from your own ideas the relevant values that should be applied to looking after other people?
- Imagine you are 78 years old, arthritic, and about to move into a home. What rules would you write for the staff of the home? Create your own Resident's Charter.

E N V I R O N M E N T A L
F A C T O R S

We have mentioned above some of the differences that exist between settings (domiciliary, residential, hospital and day care). They exist to cater for different needs:

Domiciliary care

This is the biggest setting. More people are looked after at home than in any other place. They are also mainly looked after by infor-

mal carers, many of them supported by statutory carers who give specific services, e.g. home care assistants, district nurses, doctors and social workers. This is fine if no specialised medical care is needed which can only be done in a hospital, and the level of care needed is such that it can be given at home. If 24-hour attention is needed, then it might be better if this took place in hospital, nursing home or residential care.

The growth of domiciliary care as an option since the implementation of NHS and Community Care Act 1990 has led to a rapid growth in the development of private domiciliary care agencies, but even these cannot always meet the demands made on them. They often do not have enough staff available to cover the people who are asking for their services.

Residential care

This is the term used for places where people in need of care live together, either in the same building or in the same complex. It may be an old people's home, a hostel for recovering mentally ill people, or a village community for people with learning disabilities. There are also homes and hostels for people with physical disabilities.

The level of care given usually deals with the normal routines of day-to-day living, such as dressing, bathing, eating, toileting, and getting in and out of bed (remember, there will be a variety of different people with different needs).

If the client is assessed as needing residential care, a financial assessment is made and they may have to pay towards this cost. This fact often deters people who really need this type of care from applying for it. In fact, even domiciliary care services are subject to financial assessment now.

Hospital

Hospital care will be needed for a higher level of care. Hospitals provide medical treatment either as the need arises (usually in emergency situations) or by appointment after a need has been identified. When the medical need has been met, the system is that people move to another setting. This may be back home, with domiciliary care services arranged for any continuing care required. It may be on to a nursing home, or even a residential setting, if that is what the care plan dictates.

There are sometimes problems with this system, when patients are ready for discharge from hospital, and there are delays in arranging the new setting. Beds become blocked, and new patients cannot be admitted until the transfer takes place. This happens more with elders than with other groups of patients, but it also happens with people ready for discharge from psychiatric hospitals, and learning difficulties patients.

Sometimes the reason is a skills shortage in making assessments; there are never enough community occupational therapists (COTs), and in some areas, a waiting list for assessments by a social worker.

Nursing homes

Nursing homes give general nursing care, such as changing dressings and giving injections and other treatments. They can also look after people who are totally helpless and need to have everything done for them. Continuing care and aftercare is provided, rather than the high-tech medical care available in hospitals. Nevertheless, nursing homes must by law have a qualified nurse on duty at all times (unlike residential homes, which do not have to follow this requirement).

Day care

This is a service which can support domiciliary services and is arranged for all client groups, but not necessarily always in the same area.

Day centres including luncheon clubs are popular for elders. They are usually open for five days a week, but an increasing number are now open for seven days a week. This does not mean that the same people attend every day, or indeed for all of the day. Attendance is arranged to suit individuals and their carers, and may be for one, two three or more days a week, or for some half-days a week.

Nurseries and playgroups are a form of day care for children, and the same is true of them. The same children may not be there all the time, but for parts of a day, or some days a week to suit the parents.

Day centres for people with physical disabilities, or people recovering from a mental illness are also to be found in many towns. Hospitals may also have *day hospitals* for mentally ill people, or *day wards* for giving minor surgery or diagnostic tests.

LOCATION

Whether people live in the country (a rural location), or in a town (an urban location) can make a difference to the services they receive. The availability and cost of transport can become a major issue.

The range of provision is likely to be less in rural locations than in urban ones. The majority of the big hospitals are situated in or near to the big towns, where most of the population live, and so most of the need arises. The same is true of voluntary organisations, particularly local branches of national organisations. They will have offices

---

**Accessible Transport
Maybury Dial-A-Ride**

This is a door-to-door Dial-a-ride service for people who are unable to use ordinary buses due to disability. In order to use the service you will need to join the Dial-a-Ride Club, but membership is free.

Phone:	(01234) 567890
Address:	Maybury Dial-a-Ride Club, c/o The County Transport Co-ordinator, Recton Business Centre Mill Lane, Maybury
Area covered:	All the urban areas
Operating hours:	9.30 a.m.–6.00 p.m. Monday, Tuesday, Thursday, Saturday
When to book:	9.00 a.m.–1.00 p.m. Monday to Saturday, the day before you want to travel
Single Fare:	£1 adults
Concessions:	50p for holders of disabled, senior citizens or blind persons' bus passes, also children
Escorts:	Charged at appropriate fare
Vehicles used:	Wheelchair accessible minibuses

Figure 6.11   *A Dial-a-Ride transport advert*

and other premises in the larger towns, but rarely in rural locations.

Rural villages may have a GP surgery or health centre. There could also be a residential or nursing home. They have the added advantage that property prices are often lower than they would be in towns, and staff cheaper to employ. Many old manor houses have been converted to residential care homes; they are large by today's standards, and not suitable any more for a single family to live in.

Most villages have a playgroup, but there is unlikely to be day care other than for children. Some local authorities and some voluntary organisations are meeting needs by a converted bus or coach which travels to rural locations and gives a limited service for a few days a week where there is a demand.

Transport

Hospitals use the ambulance service to bring people in to them who cannot get there by other means. Social services have transport facilities, and will collect people and return them home as part of a care plan.

Both the NHS and local authorities can help with fares for public transport in certain circumstances. Many places also have a Dial-a-bus service for disabled people which can be used for going to day care or out-patients appointments, as well as going shopping or for leisure purposes. These are useful for people who live in isolated locations where even the village is a distance to travel.

Domiciliary services

As well as the problem of transporting clients and patients to the care settings (which is yet another organisational constraint), there is the reverse problem of providing domiciliary services. Some staff such as HCAs can be recruited locally, but others will probably have to travel out from the town (such as district nurses, health visitors, hospital consultants).

Overall, this means that it is more expensive to provide most types of care in rural areas than it is in the towns. The exception is with residential care, where larger properties are available in rural areas at less cost than in urban areas, and staff may be employed at cheaper rates of pay, as there are fewer job opportunities available, and there are fewer travel to work costs involved.

HUMAN AND PHYSICAL RESOURCES

As you will have noticed from the GNVQ course so far, care relies primarily on people (human resources), and secondarily on physical resources such as buildings and equipment.

Human resources

Human resources required for care differ with individual need. Parents are fully able to cope with large families with no outside help in normal circumstances. In abnormal circumstances such as illness or other family crises, then a doctor or other care staff (nurses, social workers, etc.) may be called upon.

In our society, teachers and health professionals are involved as normal routine in educating and ensuring the health of children (e.g. immunisations, health screening, dental care). This is required by law, and does not have to be requested. The investment in personnel to cover this requirement for all children is a major expenditure from taxation.

Activity 15

Read the following care plan, and identify the human resources involved in implementing it.

CASE STUDY 12 – CARE PLAN

Mr and Mrs Hallwood are both in their sixties. Mr Hallwood has had a stroke which affected his speech and mobility. He retired at 59 because of this, and has a pension from his work plus the state pension to live on. Mrs Hallwood has a weak heart and cannot walk far or exert herself for long without becoming breathless. They have a package of care to support them in their own home. A social worker and a community occupational therapist worked together to design this package of care.

Daily

08.15   A home care assistant calls to help Mr H get out of bed, wash, dress, and go to the toilet. When he is safely downstairs in his riser chair, the HCA leaves Mrs H to see to the breakfast and moves on to the next visit.

11.00   One of three neighbours who take it in turns to visit will call in to have coffee and biscuits with them. This gives the Hallwoods some outside company, and also acts as a check visit to see that everything is in order. They will also do any shopping or collect their pension if asked.

12.30   Meals on wheels are delivered; Mrs H has the oven ready to warm them up ready to eat. She then cuts up any large items in the meal (such as meat), and puts the plate on a tray with a non-slip mat for her husband. He then uses large-handled utensils to eat it with.

15.00   A volunteer from the neighbourhood centre calls in to see that everything is alright, and have a cup of tea with them.

17.30   Mrs H's sister calls in on her way home from work to help get their evening meal ready. She will also take laundry away and do that if it is needed.

22.15   The evening HCA calls to put Mr H to bed. There is also an alarm call system fitted to the phone. Both Mr and Mrs Hallwood wear a necklace with an alarm button on it which will activate the phone. The system is connected to a control centre, and they can send help immediately if called.

Weekly

On *Sundays*, Mrs H's sister and her husband collect the Hallwoods and take them out for an hour or two and give them Sunday dinner.

On *Wednesday* afternoons, a volunteer driver collects them for a social afternoon for elders at a Community Centre.

The GP pays a routine visit every other *Tuesday*.

A visiting hairdresser comes when requested, and so does a chiropodist.

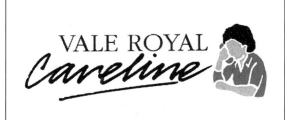

Figure 6.12   *An increasing number of companies offer care services for people in their own homes*

Physical resources

We have already mentioned that these include buildings and transport. They also include a great many other things which are not necessarily quite as expensive.

Activity 16

- Read through the above care plan again, and see how many aids to daily living you can identify in the Hallwood household.
- Collect as many magazines and newspapers as you can cope with, and find all the advertisements for items which can help people with disabilities. Examples are reproduced in Figures 6.13 and 6.14.
- Get in touch with some of the companies advertising physical aids and ask for a copy of their catalogue. Boots the Chemist also have a catalogue of items for disabled people, which can be obtained from their larger stores.
      There are also other specialists suppliers, see Fig. 6.15.

Activity 17

Draw a plan of one floor of your own home, or a part of your school or college (example shown in Fig. 6.16)

GLIDE UPSTAIRS ON A STANNAH STAIRLIFT.

Hello, Stan here. With a Stannah Stand-on Stairlift, you can glide upstairs in a standing or sitting position, safely and smoothly. For your free information pack, complete and return the coupon or call us today.

When your thoughts turn to stairs turn to Stannah.

Phone FREE (0800) 715300 or return the coupon below.

Please complete and return to: Stannah Stairlifts Limited, Dept 8056, FREEPOST, Andover, Hants SP10 3BR.

Are you enquiring for your Household ☐   A relative living elsewhere ☐

Name

Address

Postcode   Tel

Stannah *Stairlifts*

Figure 6.13   *This company offers physical aids for people who have difficulty in getting up and down stairs*

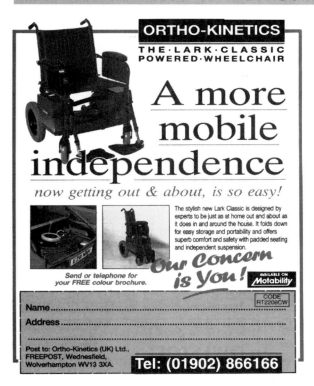

Figure 6.14 *There are many companies which design and produce wheelchairs*

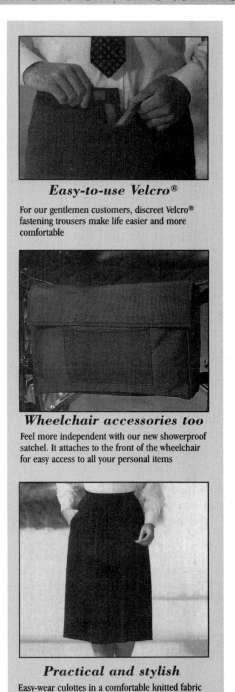

Easy-to-use Velcro®

For our gentlemen customers, discreet Velcro® fastening trousers make life easier and more comfortable

Wheelchair accessories too

Feel more independent with our new showerproof satchel. It attaches to the front of the wheelchair for easy access to all your personal items

Practical and stylish

Easy-wear culottes in a comfortable knitted fabric

Figure 6.15 *Examples of specially adapted clothes and accessories*

Put in the furniture as well as the doorways and any fitted cupboards or kitchen equipment. Using the brochures and catalogues you have collected, redesign the area you have drawn to make it more suitable for people with a disability.

Some points to bear in mind are:
• Would a ramp replace steps?
• Is a lift needed?
• Are the doorways wide enough to take a wheelchair?
• Are there any places where grab-rails would be of help?

It is worth remembering that while only about five per cent of disabled people need to use wheelchairs, when a place is made wheelchair accessible, it also helps people with poor

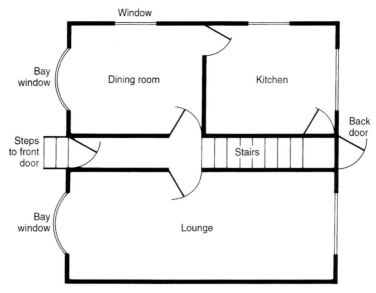

Figure 6.16   *Ground floor of house (see Activity 17)*

mobility, and parents with children in prams and pushchairs.

Write a report to explain why you have done whatever you have done.

CASE STUDY 13

Elizabeth Shah resides in a residential home in the town where she has always lived. She even went to school with some of the other residents. Elizabeth shares a room with one of them. She herself has diabetes and arthritis, failing sight, and poor hearing. She can walk a short distance, but uses a wheelchair most of the time. She needs help with dressing, toiletting, bathing, cutting up her food and with her medication.

There are 29 other elders living in the same building.

Activity 18

 Read through Case Study 13.
- How many staff do you think will be required to look after the 30 people in this residential home?
- What would their job titles be?

When you have written down what you think, do some research and find out what the actual requirements are. This may mean telephoning or writing to local residential homes, or inviting a representative from one to come to school or college and tell you about it. There may also be some resources in your school or college library to help you.

Summary

This chapter helps you build on information you have from Mandatory Units 3 and 4 by:

- examining the methods used to assess care needs, and trying them out via role play and the use of case studies provided

- looking at how needs can be met in different types of care setting, and how environmental factors can affect the delivery of care
- investigating possible factors which can influence the delivery of care in different setting
- describing how assessment leads to care plans
- discussing how clients can be involved in care planning and in shaping the care environment, and how physical resources can affect the delivery of care
- describing the roles of different types of care workers, and how human resources can affect the delivery of care
- discussing the importance of care values in any context associated with care.

There are also links to Mandatory Units 1 (diets) and 2 (valuing individuals).

7

CREATIVE ACTIVITIES IN CARE SETTINGS

AIMS AND OBJECTIVES

The aim of this chapter is to explore the concept of human creativity, and to examine the role and value of creativity in health care. By the end of the chapter you should be able to:

- understand the value of creative expression at all stages of the life span

- recognise the practical expression of your own creativity

- identify a range of creative activities

- discuss the practicalities of planning, running and evaluating creative activities for individuals and groups

- discuss the value of creative activity to different client groups

- plan and carry out a creative activity with an individual or a group

Creativity and the individual

CASE STUDY 1 – THE SAND PIT

Four-year-old Katie was crouched in the corner of the nursery sand-pit, intently stirring, sifting and digging. She picked up the red plastic sand-castle bucket, and started to fill it. As the sand neared the top, it was patted well down and the surface smoothed off. She thought for a moment and looked about her, and then took the little yellow spade she had used to fill the bucket, and pushed it into the sand so that it stood up. Another brief pause for inspiration, and this was followed by a stick, a long orange plastic cone and two lolly sticks, all driven firmly into the sand so that they stood up like stakes. Katie then brushed the drying sand off her hands, got up, took a pace backward and began to sing:

Happy birthday to you
Happy birthday to you

Happy birthday Mr Andrew
Happy birthday to you

'Mr Andrew, you've got to come and blow the candles out.' Mr Andrew came over and duly obliged. 'No, no! You've got to blow harder!' Mr Andrew blew harder. 'No, no! You've got to blow them ALL OUT!' Suddenly tumbling to what was required, Mr Andrew blew extremely hard, at the same time tipping the bucket from underneath, emptying its contents back into the sand heap. This appeared to be a most satisfactory outcome for Katie, who immediately started to gather her implements together again and make another identical birthday cake, but this time for Miss Margaret. Miss Margaret likewise fell in with what was required, after which the sandplay suddenly lost its appeal, and Katie went off to do other things.

Before we even begin to think about using creative activities with health care clients, we need to develop a clear understanding of what creativity is, and the role it plays in the health and well-being of us all. In practice, we need to take a good look at what creativity means to us, and the way it expresses itself in our lives as individuals and as members of groups.

WHAT IS CREATIVITY?

We probably all have a vague mental image of what creativity is, what it 'looks like'. But it often isn't until we come to trying to define creativity that we discover what a hard task it is. Why not give it a try – before your own thoughts and ideas are influenced by the thoughts and ideas that are expressed further on in this chapter? Take ten minutes to write a definition of creativity. Then share your definition with others in your group; are they all different or do they have things in common? Can you come up with a combined effort that gets to the heart of the matter?

If you have found this a difficult task, you are not alone. Many 'experts' in the fields of psychology and education struggle with the concept too. However, most authorities are in agreement with certain common ideas, and we will examine these below.

First of all, it is perhaps helpful to look at what creativity is *not*. Creativity is not just craftwork, nor is it to be understood simply in terms of the things we do with our hands. Creativity is not necessarily anything to do with being artistic, nor is it the privilege of the 'gifted' few.

Creativity is much broader, much richer, much more profound than these superficial concepts. So what *is* it? Let us begin by saying that creativity is something that is absolutely central to the order of life. It is the process of bringing something new to birth; bringing into being something that has never before existed in quite the same shape or form. All the achievements and advances of human history, from the wheel and the crossbow to the jet engine and the computer, are the product of the creativity and ingenuity of men and women.

Creativity lies within the potential of every human individual. Not everyone has the ability needed for crossbow or computer, but all have the *potential* to 'give birth' to innovation and originality in some fashion. Without creativity, the survival of humankind is threatened, and civilisation cannot progress: creativity is the essence of life itself. If we ignore it, we lose something critical to our understanding of life and growth. Much learned material has been written by scholars over the years; we will look very briefly at the work of three, in order to help us understand the concept.

1 **Dr Carl Rogers:** author of the 'person-centred' approach to psychology and psychiatry. He states that any act of creativity must result in a *new* and *tangible product* which has developed from the individual's relationship with the world around him. In other words, creativity is not just a new idea, but one which is fashioned into something that may be experienced, seen, touched or heard.

2 **Rollo May**, a psychoanalyst, has suggested that the true creative act is an *encounter* of intense commitment between a person and his environment, e.g. between painter and landscape, climber and mountain, baker and yeast, lover and beloved.

3 The psychiatrist **Erich Fromm** suggests that creativity is the product of four 'inner' conditions.
   - the ability to be puzzled, to wonder, to be surprised

- the capacity for single-minded concentration, by which he means being totally absorbed in the here and now
- the ability not to avoid life's conflicts, but to accept them as the source of wondering and deal with them out of our own capacities
- the ability to let go of the past, in order to embrace the unknown future by relying upon our own creative potential

Before we put these theories into practice, we should note Rogers' caution that creativity can only flourish where individuals and their products are *valued* for what they are, where there are no strings attached and no moral judgements passed. If a young person is ridiculed for the unusual way in which he expresses himself, his creative spark may be smothered and possibly extinguished.

In summary then, creativity is the capacity to meet and engage fully with our environment, making of it something that is uniquely our own. It has been described as the natural, in-born impulse of the child, surrounded on all sides by new, uncharted experiences. He cannot be other than creative as he uses his limited abilities to solve the puzzle that is the world. Those who want to retain that creativity into adulthood must hold on to the wonder and the curiosity of the young child: there must be a part of each adult that remains forever a child.

Activity 1 – Discussion

 Go back to page 210 now and re-read Case Study 1, The Sand Pit. Is it possible to link any of these thoughts and ideas with the creativity that we see expressed in Katie?
- How is Katie expressing her creativity?
- What inner resources is she drawing upon?
- How is her creativity being nourished?
- What value might this activity have had for Katie?

Activity 2

 Think for a few minutes about yourself and your own creativity, and make a brief note of:

1 a creative activity you engaged in as a child
2 a creative activity you are engaged in now
3 a creative activity you think you might engage in as an older person, perhaps when you retire

With a partner, discuss some of the following questions.
- Why did you choose to engage in these particular activities (1 and 2)?
- What personal and environmental resources did you draw upon to be able to carry them out?
- What was the result? Did you become skilled? Did you continue to pursue that activity? If you didn't, what made you give it up?
- Is there a contrast between these activities and those you think you might do in later life (3)? If so, what is the difference and why should it occur?

Activity 3

 • Come together as one large group and paint a mural. It doesn't have to be a real one; a large piece of paper on the floor or attached to the wall will do, but the larger your group, the larger your paper will need to be. Gather a variety of coloured paints or pastels and decide upon a theme. The choice is yours: you could draw something zany like a new underwater theme park, or the biggest burger in the world; or something along a more serious line, like designing a garden for disabled people, or fashion through the ages. It's up to you; let the mood take you.
- When the task is complete, take a short

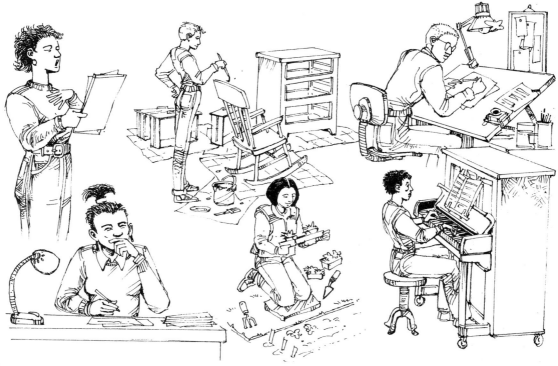

Figure 7.1   *You might have done some of these creative activities in the past – but can you imagine how you would feel if you wanted to do something, but were unable?*

break and then discuss the experience in your large group. The questions below will help you, but remember that the key issue is *your* experience of creativity in this exercise.

- What were your over-riding feelings while doing this exercise – pleasure, frustration, boredom?
- What was the reason for these feelings?
- What was the general mood of the group?
- Were you able to do as you wanted, or were you held back by others?
- Was it a project of group co-operation, or just a bunch of individuals working next to each other? Why?

- Did different roles emerge among group members? Why and how?
- How does this group exercise compare and contrast with other ways in which you express your creativity?

There are of course, no right or wrong feelings or responses in this exercise. It may be that you are unable to express your own creativity in this manner. That is unimportant. What is important is your own experience of a creative activity, and that you are able to let each new experience shape your own creative expression.

Planning creative activities

CASE STUDY 2 – THE GARDEN

The plan was to rebuild the garden. Helen, the manager of the halfway house, had been wanting to do something about it ever since she arrived. She would not have called herself a gardener, but she loved colour, beauty and order, and this garden was a junk heap, choked with the decay and neglect of years. Simon and Dave agreed. Simon was 28, struggling with a drug and alcohol problem and trying to stay out of psychiatric hospital. Dave was 20 but behaved like a 12-year old, struggling to come to terms with a childhood of abuse and neglect, and trying to stay out of prison.

Reluctantly at first, but with a growing sense of purpose and achievement, the three began their attack on the garden. It quickly took over the life of the home. Skips arrived, were filled and taken away; sledge-hammers were wielded, spades broken and rotovators hired. Plans were drawn and re-drawn, and suppertimes were dominated by discussions on whether to plant shrubs or flowers, turf or grass seed. They read seed catalogues, took trips to the garden centre and gradually the garden began to take shape.

Simon fell naturally into the role of foreman. He worked from dawn to dusk, lost weight, gained muscle and a sun-tan. He started to sleep well at night, stayed off the streets and out of the pub. Dave took orders from Simon in a way that he had never done from anyone. He got muddy and sweaty and swore at the stubborn tree stumps instead of at people. He grew in stature as a man. Indeed, he had never been treated as a man before, never known how to share and work in partnership, and had never had a job before. And Helen saw *her original ideas taking shape and bear fruit*. The garden came together; and while making new discoveries about the nature and nurture of plants, she learned too, about human relationships, about *effective care* and *good communication*.

Simon, Dave and Helen have all moved on now and gone their separate ways. The house was sold. But the garden is still there, a small living testament to friendship, co-operation and goodwill.

We have already noted that often when we consider creative activity, our minds go automatically in the direction of arts and crafts; we think of a picture, a sculpture, a tapestry, a wood carving, etc. But we have seen too that creativity is something much more than mere handiwork. If we allow our understanding of creative activities to be confined in such a way, we limit our usefulness in the practical work of caring for others.

Go back to the definition we arrived at in the previous section on page 212. Surely the act of creativity is any action to which we commit ourselves fully, with the intention of making an impact upon our environment?

The letter that you write to a friend describing a holiday or sharing a problem: isn't this a creative act? The party with a 'This is your life' spot that you organise for your grandmother's 80th birthday: isn't this using your skills and your personality to construct something tangible from the environment that has never existed before? And what about the hospital visit to the miserable old next-door neighbour who always shouts at children, the gift of fruit that you bring and the squeeze of the hand: isn't this a creative act too, a bringing to birth of a new relationship? Don't be limited in your thinking by the 'art and craft' model. Creativity is that which *you* bring to birth, be it song, joke, event, relationship or tomato plant, which bears the stamp of your own uniqueness.

We must bear these things in mind as we plan creative activities. We may of course be planning activities for use on a one-to-one basis with an individual. More often in care settings, time and money restrictions dictate

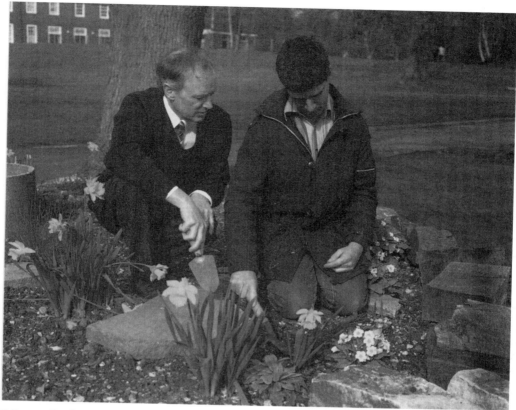

Figure 7.2   *Gardening can be creative and therapeutic for all kinds of people*

that we work with groups, both large and small. Either way, the principles upon which we base our planning remain much the same, though the preparation and practice may be quite different.

Activity 4 – Discussion

Refer back to Case Study 2, The Garden. Re-read it, and discuss in groups the issues raised by the following questions:

- Where did the creativity lie in this project?
- What skills and abilities were required of each individual to undertake this task?
- What group interaction skills were required?
- In addition to those already listed, what other benefits might have come out of this project?

- What resources would the group need to have drawn upon in order for the project to take place?
- How might Helen have built upon this activity to develop Simon and Dave's skills and self-esteem?

COMMENT

A closer study of the issues involved in the garden project gives us some useful pointers about running creative activities. It is perhaps helpful to think in terms of *preparation, practice* and *evaluation*. You may find the following checklists a practical guide as you plan and organise creative activities yourself.

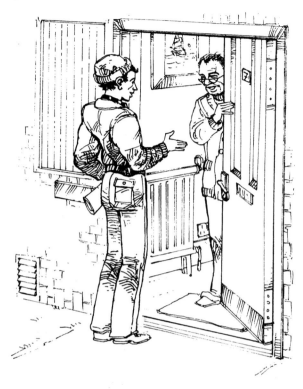

Figure 7.3   *A visit to an elderly neighbour might be their only contact with the outside world*

Preparation

- What activity is the personal preference of the client(s)?
- What is the aim of the activity?
- What skills are required for participating in this activity?
- What skills are required for running this activity?
- Is the activity appropriate to the disability?
- Is the activity appropriate to the age of the client(s)?
- Is there an appropriate setting in which the activity can take place?
- Is there an appropriate time at which the activity can take place?
- How long should each activity session be?
- Is it a one-off, or a series of activity sessions?

- Is there enough money to finance the activity?
- Are appropriate materials available?
- In a group setting, is there a compatible mix of clients?
- Are there sufficient helpers to enable the activity to run smoothly?

Practice

- Are you allowing the client(s) to do as much for themselves as possible?
- Do the challenges of the activity match the skills of the client(s)?
- What is the overall mood of the client(s)?
- Are you working alongside the client(s)?
- Are you offering appropriate praise and encouragement?
- In a group setting, are you distributing your time and attention equally?
- Are you helping clients interact with one another?
- Are you able to share out tasks between helpers?

Evaluation

- Have you discussed the activity with the client(s)?
- Have you discussed the activity with your helpers?
- Did the activity run smoothly?
- Were aims achieved?
- Was the pace of the activity appropriate for the client(s)?
- Were the materials adequate and appropriate for the activity?
- Were personal relationships comfortable?
- How were interruptions/disruptions handled?
- Were clients satisfied with their achievements?
- Did helpers work as a team?
- What improvements would you make next time?

- Should the activity continue for further sessions, or is it time to stop?
- Are there areas in which you need outside help — perhaps from a senior staff member?

There are odd occasions when a creative activity will occur spontaneously, without planning; an individual will suddenly get a creative urge and decide that there is something that they want to do; a group will respond to the bright idea of another. Often, such activities are very successful and rewarding for the person(s) concerned, who may be carried along in a wave of enthusiasm.

More often though, particularly in care settings where people have special needs, carers themselves have to start the momentum for creative activity, sometimes in the face of boredom, disinterest and disability. Where this is the case, *enthusiasm, commitment, innovation* and indeed *creativity* is required on our part. The more damaged the client(s), the harder the task usually is for us, and the more attention we need to give to preparation, practice and evaluation. If you have prepared well, and learned from previous evaluations, it is very likely that your session will run well.

- Never neglect preparation; always carry out an evaluation.

Don't worry if an occasional session goes badly; we all make a mess of it from time to time. People are unpredictable, and there are times (in group activities particularly) when all the planning in the world won't prepare you for this. So if it has gone wrong, don't worry too much. The key is to look back and understand why. If you can do this, and make an honest review of your own strengths and weaknesses, you will know what to do next time. It is the person who can't see, or doesn't take time to understand problems, who does damage.

Anyone can run creative activities, but not everyone can run them well. Running activities (particularly in groups) is skilled work, so you should take time to learn.

Activity 5

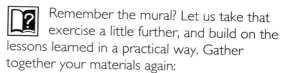 Remember the mural? Let us take that exercise a little further, and build on the lessons learned in a practical way. Gather together your materials again:

- The task is to plan, run and evaluate a group activity in which a group of adolescents are going to paint a mural on the wall in the residential facility where they live.
- Split into groups of about six or seven. In each group, two or three of you are to take the role of activity leaders; the rest take the role of teenage girls and boys.
- Activity leaders — discuss how you are going to run this activity. You have already experienced it for yourself and will therefore be aware of some of the tensions that you will be likely to meet. Don't forget, this is a 'real' mural on a 'real' wall, so it's up to you to ensure that the job is done properly.
- Teenagers — get together and decide upon the individual roles you might take. You might base the role on somebody you know, or perhaps on a difficult time in your own life. Your behaviour might be challenging, withdrawn, over-active or just plain silly (but don't make things so difficult for the leaders that the activity doesn't go at all!).

When the task is complete, stop, take a break and *evaluate* the session:
- Each should contribute their own experience of the group — how it felt, whether it was a positive growing experience, or a negative, constraining one.
- Concentrate particularly on the issues of planning, preparation and handling.
- What went well; what was good about it?
- What were the weaknesses?

- What would you change if you did another activity with the same group?

Activity 6

Run this session through again, with participants reversing roles. This time, introduce some different issues into the scenario by making it a task for a group of physically handicapped people. In this instance, the 'clients' each need to simulate a different disability:

- You might have one person in a wheelchair, another on crutches.
- A blindfold will simulate blindness, or your local RNIB may have available for loan, opaque-lensed spectacles which reproduce visual problems.
- Other simple ploys include tying one arm behind the back (stroke), ear plugs or mufflers (hearing impairment), joint braces (arthritis), thick rubber gloves (poor hand function).

Aside from the nature of the handicap, the task is the same. If you are fed up with the mural theme, try something else; but whatever you decide upon, it should be a group task, not just individuals working together in isolated projects.

COMMENT

To get the maximum benefit from these activities, it is important that everyone has the chance to experience what it is to organise and to be organised. Ensure that after each session you mark the end of the role-play, and make a point of coming out of role. Sometimes people can get very caught up in the role they are playing, and it is important that feelings and happenings that occurred during the role-play are not carried over into 'real life'. You could each announce your letting go of the role and return to self, or it may be a good idea to take a short coffee-break. Then, when you come to discussion, you should be able to look back *objectively* and *unemotionally*.

Allow sufficient time to deal with issues raised; your discussion is as important as the role-play itself.

Activity 7

In small groups of three or four, devise an afternoon programme of creative activities for an elderly persons' day centre that meets five days a week.

- Imagine that you are a group of volunteers, taking it in turns to help out on weekday afternoons during the summer holiday season when the staff team is short.

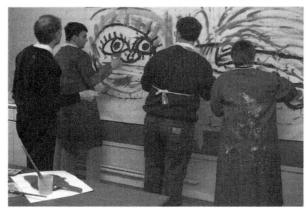

Figure 7.4   *Painting a mural together can be fun, and a useful exercise in group co-operation*

- The manager of the day centre has asked for ideas and suggestions.
- Draw up a weekly timetable of afternoon activities.
- Don't be bothered by issues of who might be able or available to conduct these activities – just brainstorm ideas.
- Try and offer two or three choices of activity each afternoon, which cover as broad a range of skills as possible – physical, social, intellectual, etc.

As an alternative, you may wish to carry out this activity as an individual written assignment, in which you offer a rationale for the activities you have selected.

The contribution of creative activities to care settings

CASE STUDY 3 – THE ART GROUP

Mrs Gregory never spoke. Or at least, she had never been known to speak in the two years she had been resident in the old people's home. She did make a sort of grunting noise to express extreme feelings though, a sort of a 'harumph'. But mostly she was quiet, and spent her time wandering about on her own, up and down the corridors and in and out of other residents' bedrooms.

This was the first time we had managed to persuade her to come along and join the weekly art group. Most people were doing block printing on this occasion, using cut vegetables, polystyrene, modelling clay and the like. As Mrs Gregory seemed unwilling to initiate any action, a carer painted some colour on to a shape and placed it into her hand. Very tentatively, Mrs Gregory placed the shape on the paper, then again, and again. In the half-hour she was there that first session, she completely covered four sheets of paper.

Over the weeks that followed, Mrs Gregory attended regularly. She would never draw free-hand, but loved to use colour on designs that were sketched for her. She would become engrossed, applying fine stroke after fine stroke, sometimes taking an hour over one petal or leaf. She started to smile and engage eye contact; she became aware of other members of the group, looking at what they were doing and nodding appreciatively.

After about eight weeks we had our usual session one Wednesday, and had finished and cleared away. About to make my way home, I happened to pass Mrs Gregory in the corridor. 'Bye, Mrs Gregory. See you next week.' Mrs Gregory put out her hand and grasped my sleeve to stop me passing her by. Her other hand came across and folded around mine, and she looked into my face. 'Thank you my dear,' she said, 'It does help to pass the time.'

Thus far, we have looked at what creativity is, and how we run creative activities. In this section we consider:

1 Why do we do creative activities?
2 What is their value to us as individuals or as groups?
3 What is their value in care settings?

If it seems odd that such an important matter is left until last, this is because we cannot fully appreciate the role and value of creative activities until we have understood and experienced them for ourselves. If you have carried out the earlier activities, you will by now have a fairly clear idea of their value in your own daily life and experience, and you will have started to think through their meaning for others.

There are, of course, no easy answers to the question 'Why are creative activities important?', because every person is unique, and experiences the world in a unique fashion. Therefore the value of creative activities is subjective; it will be *perceived* differently by each individual.

For this reason, we need to be cautious and sensitive in our planning for creative activities in care settings. It is no good planning activities, however beneficial they might seem to the carer, and then wondering why half the intended client group won't participate, or why there is a mood of indifference or reluctance. The key to the effective selection and running of creative activities is *know your client*.

This may sound simple, but it isn't. Getting to know those with whom we work takes time and effort on our part, particularly if those people do not seem interested in getting to know us. So,

• talk to your clients
• work alongside them
• ask their opinions and advice
• above all, observe.

It may be, of course, that for reasons of disability, your clients are not able, or may not wish to share themselves with you. In such a case, all you can really do is to observe, but you should also talk to those who know them well: family, friends, professionals.

Sometimes we come across a client about whom nothing is known, e.g. an elderly person who has lived alone, without family or friends. They arrive in hospital, nursing or residential home, possibly because of an infectious illness which has made them confused, and almost nothing is known about their past history, personality, skills or interests. In instances like these, we have no choice but to work in the dark, by trial and error. This lack of information should not stop us from trying to engage our client in activities, it just means that we need to work with an even greater *sensitivity* and *empathy*.

So we perhaps need to emphasise here that any given creative activity will have a *different value for each individual engaging in it.* The greater our *knowledge* and *understanding* of our client, the more effective we are likely to be in selecting appropriate activities. For example, cooking is a creative activity which is used in many care settings, but its role and its value will differ from setting to setting and client to client.

1 In the young child, it will have a developmental purpose. It encourages the child to explore textures, smells and tastes, and helps their movement and coordination.

2 In the person physically handicapped by a stroke, there will be a re-learning and adapting process, as the person discovers anew how to hold the mixing bowl still for cake-making, or the potato for peeling, when only one hand is working properly.

3 For the elderly person who is losing touch with the outside world because of a dementing process, the value of cooking will lie in its power to stimulate old memories and past experiences. Familiar smells and tastes can bring back good memories. Preparing familiar dishes can awaken dormant skills and knowledge.

4 For people with learning difficulties, its value might be as a preparation for independent living, as they get to grips with the complexities of good nutrition and budgetting after years of having meals cooked for them in institutions.

5 For the young woman with an eating

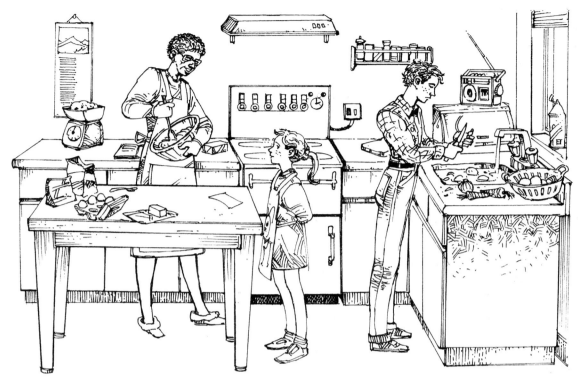

Figure 7.5   *The value of cooking as a creative activity will differ from client to client*

disorder, it might provide a way for talking through problems.

6 For the withdrawn teenager, it might be a non-threatening means of encouraging conversation, friendship and socialising.

7 For the retired person, it might have a purely social or leisure function.

8 For the young wife and mum, hospitalised with depression, it might be a means of re-gaining confidence and self-esteem.

9 For the young man who has not done well at school, it might be a means of qualification and career opportunity.

10 At the youth club barbecue, its aim might simply be to have fun.

At face value, cooking is an ordinary everyday activity. Most of us engage in it at some level every day without even thinking. But in the right hands, it is an activity of vast creative potential for health and well-being.

Activity 8 – Discussion

Refer back to Case Study 3 involving Mrs Gregory for a moment. Think about and talk through what might have been the value for this lady, of participating in the art activity. The questions below might assist your discussion.

• The key question here is not so much 'Why did she speak to me?' but 'Why had she never spoken to anyone else?'

• Why did she spend so much time wandering apparently aimlessly?

• What might have made her agree to give the art group a try?

- What was the art doing for her?
- How might staff have built upon this discovery to encourage further communication and participation?

COMMENT

ℹ️ This small scenario highlights one other important factor in creative activities which we need to deal with before we leave the subject, the *care setting* itself.

THE IMPORTANCE OF CREATIVITY IN CARE SETTINGS

Care settings are as different as the individuals whom they exist to serve. Each is unique, possessing both positive and negative qualities, strengths and weaknesses. It has to be acknowledged with regret that there are care settings where the value of creative activities is neither recognised nor understood. There are settings where, no matter how skilled and committed *you* might be in carrying out creative activities with clients, your efforts will not be supported, and may be stifled or even sabotaged. This can be simply a matter of staff shortage and lack of time. Alternatively, such a lack of concern may be rooted in long-standing negative attitudes, which can stem from:

- inadequate training/experience.
- a nursing model of care which emphasises physical needs.
- conflicts between staff engaged in 'heavy and dirty' tasks such as dealing with incontinence, and those engaged in 'nice and easy' creative activities.
- a rigid hierarchy in staff structure which does not encourage team communication.

We need to remember too, that many care settings are institutional in nature: that is, they are large and somewhat impersonal and quite unlike the small, personal home and family to which most people aspire or belong. Such environments impose their own stresses and strains by their very structure, and so most care settings are far from ideal. As care workers, we can choose to carry out our own creative activities here or there, in the home or outside it, in this club or that group, because the facilities are better here, or the teaching is better there. The person in care rarely has such a choice.

So carers who organise creative activities in care settings, need to recognise that the work environments will often not be ideal, and may set limits on *what* we are able to do and *how* we are able to do it. We are always likely to be working under certain constraints, but perhaps we can use these tensions to give us a greater empathy with our clients, for they are dealing with the same tensions, in addition to the problem of coping with their handicap.

Planning and organising creative activities in care settings is skilled work, requiring interpersonal relationships rather than in the practical expertise of art and craft. You may be a brilliant artist, or a skilled craftsman, yet quite unable to lead others into a rewarding experience of creative activity. There are three qualities that make an effective organiser of creative activities; the ability:

- to know yourself
- to know your client
- to know your environment

A simple formula, but one which involves a complex range of personal and inter-personal skills. The skills of *listening*, *observing* and *interacting* which contribute to these qualities do not come quickly or easily; there are no courses in personal integrity. They are gained over the course of time and experience, not in the classroom nor at the examination desk, but in the unpredictable and challenging arena of personal care. If this is an area in which you want to develop, the best thing you can do is to get out there and start doing. Organising activities can be demanding work, but there is nothing more rewarding than witnessing the growth of *self-esteem*, *competence* and *personal fulfilment* in clients in whom you have encouraged creative expression. This in fact is no less than a demonstration of your very own creativity. You are, in the terms of our original definition, making of your environment something that is uniquely your own. Your commitment, your enthusiasm, your empathy, are bonding with the people, the structures and the circumstances of the caring environment to bring forth something altogether new: new qualities, new capacities, new confidences, new relationships. Creativity, indeed, is at the heart of true healing.

Activity 9

 In your large group, take each of the following care settings in turn and think of the types of creative activity which you think might be suitable in such situations.

- A playgroup for the under fives.
- A young mums' coffee morning.
- A Darby and Joan club for the elderly.
- A group home for people with learning difficulties.
- A stroke club.
- A job club for the unemployed.
- A youth club for teenagers.
- A women's refuge.

Now look at the activities you have identified for each setting and ask yourselves what you would want these creative activities to achieve for the people concerned.

COMMENT

For Activities 9 and 10, your group will need to identify a number of local care settings. You have already had some examples in this chapter of the type of settings you might look for. Try and compile a list which covers as broad a range of service as possible. You probably all know of at least one or two; contact your local library, social services department or volunteer bureau for more ideas.

Activity 10

Each member of the group should make a short visit to two contrasting settings. Talk to the staff and the clients, observe the surroundings, get involved with what is going on, and above all have an awareness of the 'feel' of the place. When all your visits have been made, come together as a group (or in groups of seven or eight if you are a large class). Fill in a table such as Table 7.1, with details of the information you have picked up. When all your information is collected compare and contrast the different settings and see what general conclusions you reach.

The amount of information you can pick up on a short visit is limited, but sometimes the brief impression on an outsider is a better indicator of the true quality of care than the opinions of the insider who is working in the same environment day in and day out. Most places have a 'feel' about them and it is important to be sensitive to that impression, and to wonder why it should be this way. We must however, guard against sitting in moral judgement over any particular care unit. Care settings are usually the product of a long and complex history of personal, professional and political pressures which are not the business of the casual visitor. Our task is simply to observe and to understand.

Table 7.1   Contrasting different aspects of care settings

Centre	Group Home 2 Cherry Close	PHAB Club	Mayflower Nursing Home
Client Group	4 adults with learning difficulties	Physically handicapped and able-bodied	Elderly, mentally and physically infirm
Staff	RMNs from local hospital call daily	Two SW One OT	Some trained nurses. Some unqualified assistants
Support Workers	One volunteer to give weekly literacy class	Several (able-bodied help handicapped)	None evident. One visitor helping mother eat lunch
Building	Three bedrooms, semi detached house Nice decor	Church hall. Quite modern. Good facilities	Like hospital. All white. No colour
Type of Care	As required to maintain independence	Social/recreational	Nursing and physical
Culture	Rural/village	Inner city – multi-cultural	Coastal town – retired area
Creative Activity	One lady knitting. One daily to day centre. One out. One watching TV	All sorts. Everyone occupied. Regular outings	None evident. Everyone asleep in chairs
Feel-Good Factor	OK. Quiet and subdued. Quite homely but nothing exciting	Good. Made very welcome. Enjoyed myself	Grim. Glad to get out. Felt very sad

The questions below might assist your discussion.

- Which are the settings with an above-average 'feel-good' factor?
- Do these centres have features in common which might account for this?
- Is there a link between creative activities and the 'feel-good' factor?
- Do the services to one age group appear to be better than those to another age group?
- Does any particular service appear to be better catered for overall?

- What impact does the building appear to have on services?
- What impact does the staff team appear to have on services?

Activity 11

Select a care setting from your list that is of particular interest to you, and which would be prepared to accommodate you over several visits. Your task in this final exercise is to examine a care setting in some depth, exploring

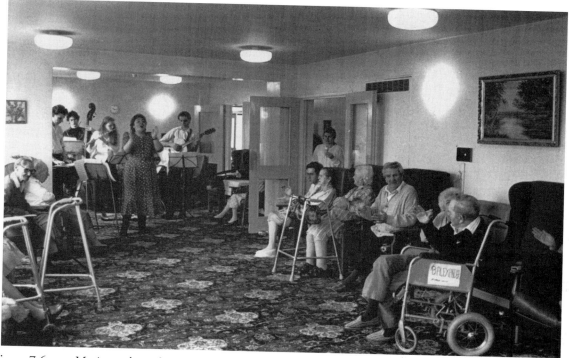

Figure 7.6   *Music can bring back memories of youth, and encourage participation*

the role and value of creative activities in that setting. Once you have obtained permission from the manager of the unit, spend as much time there as you can. Try not to clutter your first visit(s) with information gathering and note-taking. Just allow yourself to experience the life of the place. Work with the staff, work with the clients, share their meals, get to know the building, the routines. Above all, listen and observe. When you have begun to feel comfortable on the unit, decide upon one of the following projects which will enable you to carry out an in-depth study of creative activities in care settings.

PROJECT A

1 Devise a simple questionnaire, which will help you to gain information on the role and value of creative activities in your chosen setting. Use open-ended questions that encourage people to express their feelings and opinions. Avoid questions that require just a yes/no answer. You may need to think of different questions for clients and staff.

2 Using your questionnaire, interview as many people in the unit as are willing to talk to you. Don't be bound by the questionnaire; you will probably find that most people are flattered by your interest and prepared to talk freely. But in case they don't, your questionnaire gives you a bit of structure.

3 Using your information, draw out common themes and construct an essay on your findings. You might use actual quotes and specific examples to add colour to your ideas. Don't be afraid of indicating your own opinions, but make sure you clarify which are yours and which are those of the people you have interviewed.

PROJECT B

Carry out a case study on a client whom you have got to know fairly well. Concentrate on one or more creative activities in which the client is engaged, monitoring over a period of time. Ideally, you should be involved in the selection, planning, introduction and teaching of the activity, but you will have to work with whatever circumstances present themselves.

Work with the client, obtaining his/her view at all times on the selection and the carrying out of the activity. If you have a client who is not able to express his/her wishes, you will need to obtain permission for your study from the client's relations and the unit manager. As you introduce and conduct the activity, you will need to look out for visual evidence of the impact of the activity.

In your essay, you should give a pen portrait of the client (using a false name of course) and an account of the activity selected. Describe the course of the activity and indicate your own opinion of the value of the activity, as well as the client's. You may want to use the checklists in the previous section on page 216 to help structure your essay.

PROJECT C

Plan, introduce and carry out a creative activity with a group of clients in one session only. Again, you may find the earlier checklists helpful, and you will almost certainly need the advice and co-operation of the unit staff team. Write an essay on your experiences of the session, commenting in particular on the impact of the activity on the group, and on the individual members of the group.

SUMMARY

- Creativity is the capacity to engage fully with your environment (people, things, events), making of it something uniquely your own.
- All advances in the history of humankind are directly due the creativity of its members.
- The capacity for creative expression is common to all people, not just to a gifted minority.
- Creative expression is important at all stages of the human life span.
- Creative activities require sensitive recognition of the uniqueness of each individual.
- Successful creative activities require efficient planning and honest evaluation.
- Critical qualities of an effective activities organiser are the ability to know oneself, to know the client and to know the environment (the care setting).
- As far as possible, creative activities and the manner in which they are carried out, should be the choice of the client or the client group.
- Any given creative activity is likely to have a different role and value, according to the individual who is engaging in it.
- Care settings are all very different, and have a varying appreciation of, and commitment to creative activities with clients.

DEFINITIONS

Person centred approach A counselling approach in which the client is encouraged to devise his own solutions to problems.

Care setting Any geographical location in which direct health or social care is provided. Refers usually to the building in which the service operates e.g. hospital, nursing home, day centre.

Encounter   A meeting

Further Reading

Anderson, H. (ed) (1959), *Creativity and Its Cultivation.* Harper and Row.

Dynes, R. (1988), *Creative Writing in Groupwork.* Winslow Press.

Dynes, R. (1990), *Creative Games in Groupwork.* Winslow Press.

Jennings, S. (1986), *Creative Drama in Groupwork.* Winslow Press.

Campbell, J. (1993), *Creative Art in Groupwork.* Winslow Press.

Payne, H. (1990), *Creative Movement and Dance in Groupwork.* Winslow Press.

Archibald, C. (1990/1993), *Activities/ Activities II.* Dementia Services Development Centre, University of Stirling.

Briscoe, T. (1991), *Develop an Activities Programme.* Winslow Press.

Walsh, D. (1993), *Groupwork Activities.* Winslow Press.

8

PRACTICAL CARING SKILLS

AIMS AND OBJECTIVES

This chapter looks at the different places and types of care available to meet the needs of older people. When you have completed this chapter you will be able to:

- understand the different types of care available in different settings

- explain your role in supporting older people who require care

- be aware of the Community Care Act 1990, Health and Safety legislation and your responsibilities

- explain how the layout of the home and the way staff work with people affects the person's abilities

- explain your role in supporting older people who require help with physical needs

- understand how you can help people to bath, dress, eat and move around

- be aware of the importance of treating each person as an individual with physical and emotional needs

---

Types of care settings

There are many different kinds of care setting, which give various levels of care, depending on the needs of the client. An elderly person who is acutely ill, requires medical or surgical treatment, or high levels of medical care, is cared for in hospital. He or she will stay in hospital for a short period, normally a few weeks. Following treatment he or she will be discharged from hospital, and will probably return home. But some people do not recover completely and may require further assistance or ongoing nursing care, either in a home or in the community.

THE COMMUNITY CARE ACT 1990

The Community Care Act 1990 was introduced in April 1993. It has two main aims:

1 to enable people who are not acutely ill but require ongoing nursing care or help with the activities of daily living, to receive that care at home if they so wish. These activities include:
   - Maintaining a safe environment
   - Communication

- Breathing
- Eating and drinking
- Eliminating
- Personal cleansing and dressing
- Controlling body temperature
- Mobilising
- Sleeping
- Religious needs
- Social activity
- Expressing sexuality
- Wounds and dressings
- Dying
- The nurse may identify other needs

2 to prevent the costs of long-term care from continuing to rise. Social services departments (SSDs) became responsible for setting up a system to assess the needs of people requiring care and were allocated budgets to purchase that care. People who require emergency treatment, acute care or high levels of medical supervision remain the responsibility of the health authority.

Charges for community care

'Social care' is the term used for people who need nursing, residential, or care in their own homes. Social care in nursing and residential homes is paid for from social services budgets if the older person has savings of less than £16,000. (NB: this figure may rise with inflation – you should keep an eye on government legislation which might affect this.) If the person has savings of more than £16,000, he or she must pay the home's fees from savings. Any property owned must be sold to pay care home fees unless the person's husband or wife is living there.

If the older person is cared for at home the situation is slightly different, as obviously the property cannot be sold to pay for care. However, local authorities can make a charge against the property in order to recover the fees when the home is eventually sold. Some SSDs do not charge for home care; most do charge if the person's savings are over £16,000.

NURSING HOMES

Older people requiring high levels of skilled nursing care throughout a 24-hour period are often cared for in nursing homes. There are more than 5,000 nursing homes in the UK, caring for more than 220,000 older people. Nursing homes are regulated by the Registered Homes Act (1984) which lays down conditions of registration, inspection and record keeping within homes.

Homes are registered with the local health authority. A registration certificate giving details about the number and type of patients who can be cared for in the home is issued and must be displayed in the home. Homes pay an annual registration fee and the home is inspected at least twice each year. Inspection and registration officers can enter the home at any time. They may inspect records or ask the nurse in charge for information about day-to-day care within the home.

The person in charge of the home must be a registered nurse or a registered medical practitioner. Usually the person in charge is a nurse and is known as matron. The matron is required to keep certain records:

- A register of all patients admitted; including details of name, address, general practitioner, date of birth, date of discharge or death.
- A daily statement of the patient's health and condition.
- A record of staff employed must be kept at the home.
- Details of fire practices, fire alarm tests, fire procedures and action taken to remedy defects must be kept.

- Details of routine maintenance of equipment such as lifts, cookers, dryers and hoists.
- Homes are required under the Act to give written notice of death in writing to the health authority within 24 hours of a death occurring within the home.

The home must also provide:

- Adequate staff including ancillary staff
- Adequate space including day room space
- Adequate furniture, beds, screens to ensure privacy, medical and nursing equipment and facilities
- Adequate lighting, maintenance, cleanliness and decor
- Adequate fire precautions and staff training
- Adequate kitchen equipment, food and laundry facilities
- Adequate arrangements for disposal of clinical waste
- Adequate arrangements for patients to receive medical and dental services
- Adequate arrangements for the recording, safekeeping, handling and disposal of drugs
- Adequate arrangements for prevention of infection
- Adequate arrangements for occupational and recreation
- Adequate privacy
- Adequate precautions against the risk of accident

Nursing homes are required to have at least one registered nurse on duty at all times. The number of staff each home requires for each shift is agreed with the nursing home inspectorate and varies according to the size, layout and workload of the home. Care assistants work under the supervision of registered nurses within nursing homes.

Functions of a nursing home

- To provide skilled nursing care within a homely environment
- To enable older people to live life to the full, making real choices and decisions about their lives
- Enabling older people to regain independence following illness
- Enabling older people to retain existing abilities
- Providing support and help when required

CASE HISTORY I

Mrs Doris Logan suffered a stroke and was unable to care for herself. She moved to a residential home but fell fracturing her femur. She was admitted to hospital where surgeons repaired the fracture.

Mrs Logan then suffered a further stroke. Unable to walk, suffering from urinary incontinence and unable to use the left side of her body, she was transferred to a nursing home because she required skilled nursing care. Mrs Logan's nursing needs were assessed and a plan of care drawn up:

- Special shoes with a calliper were provided to enable her to begin walking again.
- Physiotherapy and walking practice enabled her to walk again using a tripod.
- The reasons why she had become incontinent were investigated and a continence promotion programme was commenced.

A few months after admission Mrs Logan was able to walk short distances with help and had regained continence. Although she still required help to carry out the activities of daily living, she was more independent and enjoyed taking part in the home's activities programme and following her own interests.

RESIDENTIAL HOMES

Residential homes provide the same kind of help which a caring relative would give. Residential homes are regulated under the Registered Homes Act 1984 Part 2. The regulations are similar to those governing nursing homes.

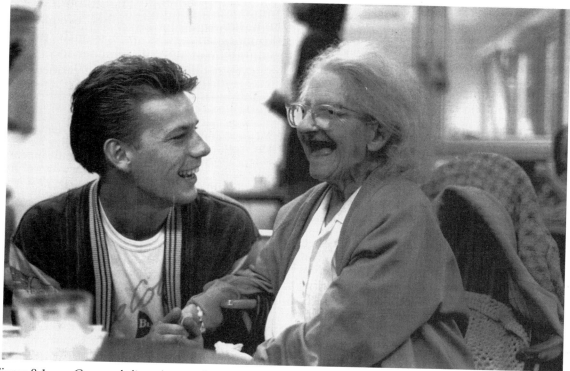

Figure 8.1   Carer and client share a joke

However, residential homes rarely employ trained nurses. In fact the Registered Homes Act forbids registered nurses working in residential homes from using their nursing skills. If older people require nursing care, e.g. dressing a leg ulcer, then this care is given by a district nurse. Residents who require high levels of nursing care for a short period may be cared for by visiting district nurses. If the person requires ongoing skilled nursing care, nursing home care may be required.

In general, residential homes employ fewer staff than nursing homes. In some homes staff may cook residents' meals, launder clothing and clean as well as providing care. Inspectors from the social services department inspect residential homes.

Functions of a residential home

- Provide support and help with activities of daily living
- Enable people to retain independence
- Provide help and support when required

DUAL REGISTERED HOMES

Dual registered homes are registered under both parts of the Registered Homes Act 1984. Normally a number of beds are registered as nursing home beds and a number as residential beds. Dual registered homes aim to enable people to remain in the home, which has become the person's own home, if condition either improves, requiring residential care, or worsens, requiring nursing care.

CASE HISTORY 2

Mrs Edith Chisholm is unmarried and has no close relatives or friends. Her neighbours have been worried about her for some time. She is becoming more forgetful, playing loud music in the middle of the night, thinking it is morning. She often goes out and forgets her keys.

She is admitted to hospital after being run over while crossing a busy road. She is found to be undernourished and suffering from dementia. Social workers visit her home, and find that it is cold, damp, dirty and unfit to live in. Nurses on the ward discover that Mrs Chisholm is very forgetful and unable to care for herself. This is confirmed by the occupational therapist who assesses Mrs Chisholm's ability to care for herself.

Mrs Chisholm admits that looking after herself has become a struggle in recent years and agrees to be transferred to a residential home. Mrs Chisholm is reassured when she becomes anxious, helped to get in and out of the bath, and provided with meals and assistance when required. She gains weight, feels much better because she has help when she needs it, and enjoys the company of others living in the home.

Only five per cent of homes are dual registered. They are inspected by both health authority and social services inspectors, pay two sets of registration fees and keep two sets of records. The government is considering abolishing the distinctions between nursing and residential homes and introducing a single category of care home.

- Dual registered homes have the same functions as nursing and residential homes.

DAY CARE

Day hospitals

Day hospitals are run by the NHS and are attended by people discharged from hospital or referred by their general practitioners. Day hospitals provide a short period of active treatment which will lead to improvement in the person's condition. Trained nurses, physiotherapists, speech therapists, occupational therapists and other professionals provide treatment and rehabilitation services. There are no charges for day hospital treatment.

CASE HISTORY 3

Mr John Morris is 76 years old. He suffered a stroke and was unable to speak or move his left side. He was admitted to hospital for treatment. During his stay he regained some movement in his left arm and leg, learned to walk with a tripod, and began to learn to speak again.

Mr Morris returned home to live with his wife. He attends a day hospital three times a week:

- Physiotherapy treatment and exercise help him to improve the strength in his muscles
- Speech therapy helps him to regain his speech
- The stroke club which is held at the day hospital gives him an opportunity to meet other people who are recovering from strokes. They discuss ways of coping with disability and attend therapy together as a group.
- Mr Morris has a bath twice weekly at the day hospital.

Day centres

Day centres are run by social services. People attending may be suffering from confusion because of diseases such as Alzheimer's disease. Many day centres lack facilities for people who find it difficult to walk or move themselves around in wheelchairs. Trained nurses are not employed: these centres are normally staffed by care assistants.

Day centres rarely offer treatments such as physiotherapy. The aim is to offer social care, providing recreational activities, company, a hot midday meal and some supervision. People who have savings of more than £8,000 may be charged for using a day centre.

CASE HISTORY 4

Mrs Janet Morris is 85 years old and widowed. She lives with her daughter Mrs Sarah Davis who is also a widow. Mrs Morris suffers from Alzheimer's type dementia and her memory is poor. She can remember the events of 50 years ago clearly but forgets to put water in the kettle before switching it on. She often forgets to eat the lunch which her daughter has prepared before going to work and sometimes forgets to go to the toilet until it is too late. Mrs Morris feels very lonely and lost when her daughter Sarah goes to work. Mrs Davis is becoming more and more anxious about leaving her mother at home alone. Both desperately want some help in coping with the situation but would not consider 'a home'.

A place at a local day centre proves to be the answer to their prayers. Mrs Morris is picked up in a minibus and taken to the centre four days every week when her daughter goes to work. Mrs Morris meets other people, enjoys a cooked lunch, takes part in a full programme of activities including Bingo. Staff at the home remind Mrs Morris to use the bathroom and ensure that she does not lose her way in the centre.

CARE WITHIN THE PERSON'S OWN HOME

Until the Community Care Act 1990 was introduced, older people requiring high levels of care had little choice but to live either in an NHS long stay elderly care unit or a nursing home. The situation has now changed dramatically; many areas offer intensive nursing support in the client's home. This is provided by district nursing teams.

Home care

Home carers care for people who require social care. Their tasks include: preparing snacks and light meals, bathing, washing and assisting older people to get in and out of bed, emptying commodes, changing inconti-

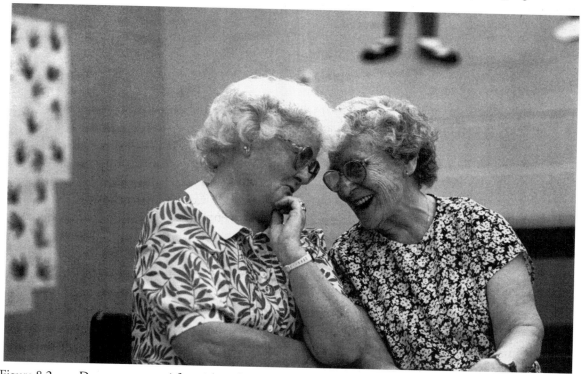

Figure 8.2   Daycentres can satisfy social needs as well as providing physical care

nence pads, and many other personal tasks. If the person requiring care is very disabled, two home carers may work together as a team to give care. Social care is means tested.

CASE HISTORY 5

Mr George Wooten has suffered from Parkinson's disease for many years. He now has difficulty in moving around and is unable to get up, wash and dress without help. He lives with his wife. Mr Wooten has four sons who live nearby with their families, and they are finding it more difficult to provide the care he requires because his condition is worsening. They request help to enable them to continue to care for Mr Wooten at home.

Home care staff are provided:

- two home carers visit each morning and help Mr Wooten to wash, dress and get out of bed
- Mrs Wooten then cares for her husband until about 3 pm when the home carers return and help Mr Wooten to bed for an afternoon nap
- One of Mrs Wooten's daughters-in-law visits and remains in the house while Mrs Wooten goes out to do some shopping or to see a friend
- She returns home to cook the evening meal and one of her sons visits to help his father get up for his meal
- Later one of Mr Wooten's sons returns and helps him to bed.

Night sitters

Some older people living with their families require 24-hour care. Relatives can become worn down through lack of sleep. Home care teams can care for the individual during the night to enable the relatives to have a rest.

CASE HISTORY 6

Mrs Alice Stewart is alert and suffers from severe arthritis. She uses a wheelchair to move around. Her husband helps her during the day but she needs help to get up to use the toilet three or four times each night. Her husband has become exhausted and finds that helping his wife at night has become a terrible strain. The home care service now provide a night sitter who attends to Mrs Stewart two nights per week while Mr Stewart relaxes and catches up on his sleep.

Activity 1

 Choose one of the care settings mentioned above, and find out all the different sorts of legislation which affect it.

Supporting social and life skills for older people

HELPING OLDER PEOPLE TO RETAIN INDEPENDENCE

People living in care homes require different amounts of help with various activities of daily living. Carers can find out about the individual's abilities from senior staff. Staff practices can help people to retain skills.

Encouraging and enabling people to do as much as possible for themselves enables them to maintain dignity and independence. Some older people who are extremely ill or disabled, will require greater levels of assistance; further information is given later in the chapter.

PHYSICAL EFFECTS OF ILLNESS

Many older people enter homes because the effects of an accident or illness mean that they can no longer manage at home. Many people enjoy life in a home where the support they require is given. Older people may require encouragement, help, support and aids to help them walk: carers should learn as much as possible about the person's abilities so that appropriate support and help can be offered.

- Diseases such as arthritis can cause pain, stiffness and difficulties in moving. There are two types of arthritis, osteo-arthritis and rheumatoid arthritis.
- Strokes cause the blood supply to the brain to be interrupted and part of the brain is starved of oxygen. People who have suffered from strokes often develop weakness or paralysis down one side of their body. Some can learn to walk with special aids. Others can learn to move around in wheelchairs and transfer to and from the wheelchair.
- Many older people suffer from a disease known as osteo-porosis, which makes bones weaker, thinner and more likely to break. Older people who fall may break thigh or hip bones. Some require special shoes as one leg is often shorter than the other after surgery. Physiotherapy and encouragement will help the individual get back on her feet.
- People who have poor eyesight find it difficult to move around. Research shows that 96 per cent of people over the age of 80 require spectacles. Regular eye tests can help detect many treatable eye conditions, and new spectacles help people to recover their confidence. Carers who discover that an individual is having difficulty seeing

should inform senior staff who can take action.

HELPING OLDER PEOPLE TO MOVE AROUND

Carers can do many things to help people in homes remain independent. However, some carers insist on doing things for the person who can do it themselves. In this case, the carer is making life more difficult. Faced with such 'help', some older people can feel that there is little point in trying and that it is better to let the staff 'get on with it'. Carers can unintentionally make older people feel useless. If a carer offers to bring a patient downstairs in a wheelchair 'because it's quicker', then the patient may soon lose the confidence and strength to come down alone. She will also lose independence and may begin to feel that she is a nuisance and a burden to staff.

CASE HISTORY 7

Mrs Juliet Johnson suffers from severe arthritis and walks with a wheeled Zimmer frame. She finds it difficult to get up from her chair. She also has difficulty getting up from the toilet.

Her doctor asked the occupational therapist to find out how she could be helped to maintain mobility and retain independence.

The occupational therapist arranged for Mrs Johnson to be provided with a special chair known as an 'Eze Rise'. This chair has a small lever; when it is pulled, the chair cushion slowly raises the person sitting in the chair and helps the person to stand up. A raised toilet seat which clips onto the toilet was also provided.

This equipment enables Mrs Johnson to remain independent.

Walking aids

There are several different types of walking aid.

ZIMMER FRAMES

These help older people who are unsteady on their feet or who lack confidence. Zimmer frames are made in a variety of heights and widths. People who do not have the strength to lift a frame off the ground are supplied with special zimmer frames which have wheels.

GUTTER FRAMES

These are specialist frames. They are often supplied to individuals who have difficulty in gripping and lifting a normal frame. People who need these frames often have severe arthritis in the arms and hands.

Individuals who use gutter frames may require the carer's help to stand up and gain their balance on the gutter frame. Sometimes the carer will walk alongside the individual.

TRIPODS

People who have suffered from strokes and have a weakness or paralysis down one side often use tripods as walking aids.

Encouraging older people to use their aids

Many people are nervous when they first receive aids, and require encouragement to use them. Staff may accompany a person on walks until they are sure that he or she is confident and safe. Some older people who use aids will always require someone to assist them. People who use aids become dependent on them and should always have these placed near them. It is easy for a carer to move an aid out of the way when settling someone in bed, and then forget to place it back within reach of the individual before leaving the room.

But, if someone is unable to reach their walking aid they may try to get up and walk without it. This can lead to a fall and the older person could suffer from a serious injury.

Gentle exercise

Using aids enables many older people to become more independent than before. Older people who use walking aids benefit from the exercise. Exercise improves the circulation to the legs and reduces the risk of swollen ankles and legs. Movement helps the bowel to work properly and the individual is less likely to become constipated. Gentle exercise such as walking may give patients who previously had no interest in food, an appetite. Overweight patients benefit from exercise, as the ability to move around and go on outings will help them to lose weight. Staff within the home have more time to spend chatting or taking part in activities with the patient as they no longer have to spend so much time helping the person move around. Family and friends may be keen to take the individual home for tea or on outings.

HELPING PEOPLE IN WHEELCHAIRS RETAIN AND REGAIN INDEPENDENCE

Some people are unable to walk even with aids and must use wheelchairs to help them move around. Patients with diseases such as multiple sclerosis or severe arthritis may need wheelchairs.

People who are unable to walk can still retain their independence if they are helped and encouraged to do so. Unfortunately many people are issued with wheelchairs which they cannot use themselves, and they must rely on others to push them. This is a great shame as many people are able to learn how to move around in their wheelchairs. There are two different types of (non electric) wheelchairs.

1 Self propelling wheelchairs have large wheels which have circular metal hand grips around them. The older person uses the hand grip to turn the wheels and push herself along. Many people are able to become independent when they get used to their wheelchairs.

Some people who have suffered from strokes have only one working hand with which to push the wheelchair. Stroke patients often request that the foot plate on the side of the body not affected by the stroke is left off. The patient then uses the unaffected leg to help steer and move the wheelchair around.

2 Some wheelchairs are designed for people who are unable to move around themselves. These chairs have smaller wheels.

Practical skills to support physical needs

MOVING AND HANDLING

The Manual Handling Regulations 1992 made employers responsible for reducing the amount of moving and handling within the workplace. Employers also have a duty:

- to assess any handling tasks
- to provide staff training
- to work out policies to reduce the risk of staff and patient injury

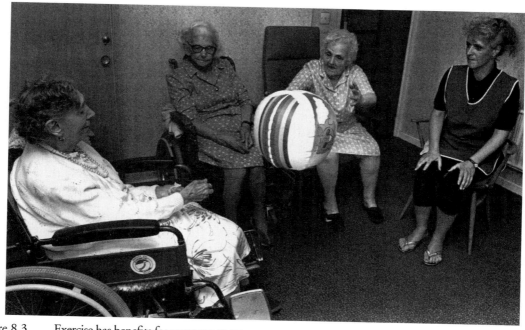

Figure 8.3   Exercise has benefits for everyone at every age

Equipment to enable staff to move patients safely must be provided. Carers should not attempt to move a person until they have received training and instruction on how to do this. Now the maximum weight one person can lift alone is 25 kg, and two people should lift a maximum of 50 kg. If a person weighs more than this and is unable to help move then a hoist should be used.

Staff responsibilities under the Regulations include following the home's moving and handling policies and using equipment provided. Each person who is unable to move without the assistance of staff should have a handling assessment completed by a senior member of staff. This will be used to form a plan of care which gives details of the methods used to move the person and equipment to be used.

Activity 2

Ask for a copy of the moving and handling assessment and the moving and handling policies used in the home you are visiting or working in.

- How are these used to plan care within the home?
- What type of aids are used in the home?

COMMENT

Include bath hoists, standing aids, hoists as well as aids which patients use to help them move around.

MAINTAINING A SAFE ENVIRONMENT

The legislation relating to a safe environment includes the Health and Safety at Work Act (1974). Under this legislation, employers and employees both have duties.

Employers

Employers who employ more than five employees have a legal duty to provide a written health and safety policy. Ask to see a copy of this – you may wish to include this in your portfolio. They must also:

- take precautions to reduce the possibility of accidents
- provide training to staff to enable them to work safely
- provide equipment to ensure the health and safety of those working and living in the home.

Employees

Staff also have responsibilities. They must:

- Comply with the home's health and safety policies
- Report hazards

Providing a safe environment within the home is very important. Older people who have poor vision or who have difficulty walking are far more at risk of injury than young healthy staff:

- An object left on the floor could easily cause an older person to stumble.
- Cleaning fluid left in a toilet might be drunk by a confused patient.
- A wet floor could cause an older person to slip and fall.
- If the light in a room does not work, this should be reported and repaired promptly to prevent the risk of injury.

Some staff worry that if the people they care for fall and injure themselves they will be blamed. In such circumstances there is the temptation to discourage people from walking or doing things for themselves in case they have an accident. It is important that staff are aware that there is no such thing as a totally safe environment. The aim of legislation is to enable older people to enjoy a good quality of life while reducing the risk of accidents. Most homes now have a policy of assessing the people who are at risk of falling – ask to see details of these policies within your home.

Activity 3

 Mr Sam Bowman has just entered the home. He is alert and fiercely independent. He has recently been registered blind but is reluctant to ask staff for help. List the possible dangers which Mr Bowman may face and how these can be avoided while independence is maintained. Some of the things you should have noted are listed in Table 8.1.

SUPPORTING OLDER PEOPLE WHO HAVE PHYSICAL NEEDS

The level of ability people living in care homes possess varies enormously. Some older people within nursing homes are very dis-abled and may require a great deal of help with the activities of daily living. The person may require a great deal of assistance or may be totally reliant on carers to eat, remain clean, provide continence care, move, prevent pressure sores developing. In such circumstances carers will be working with or under the direct supervision of a registered nurse. The individual will have a plan of care and details of the type of care given and how this is to be given will be recorded. The care plan is updated regularly by the registered nurse.

Hygiene

The people who live in care homes now had a very different life in their youth from ours today. Many did not have bathrooms or the constant supply of hot water which we now take for granted. Bathing often involved either a weekly trip to the public baths or heating up water and washing in a tin bath in front of the fire. Most of the time people washed from head to toe with a bowl of water.

Many older people enjoy bathing or show-

Table 8.1   How to avoid potential safety hazards

DANGER	ACTION
If the room is cluttered Mr Bowman could bump into furniture.	Discuss how the furniture can be arranged so he can move around safely. Then make sure that no one re-arranges the furniture without his consent as this could lead to accidents.
Could trip on any thing left on the floor, e.g. a trailing vacuum cleaner lead or a bin which is not placed in its usual position.	Make sure all staff are aware of the possible dangers and do not leave anything lying on floor.
Could trip on rugs.	If rugs are present then check that they have a non slip backing.
Could stumble or trip if packages or frames are left in the corridor or lounge.	Make sure that the corridor and lounge are kept as free of obstacles as possible. Warn Mr Bowman if he is approaching an obstacle such as another patient's frame.

ering daily but others prefer to wash each day and bath once or twice each week. It is important that carers respect the individual's wishes.

Bathing should be a pleasure, and not a rushed affair where the older person feels hurried or uncomfortable.

- Carers should ensure that the window is closed and that the bathroom is warm.
- The bath water should be at the individual's preferred temperature.
- If the older person likes to use bath oil or foam, this should be added to the water.
- Many older people require help getting in and out of the bath. You should check how much help the person requires. In many nursing homes bath hoists are used to enable older people to get in and out of baths.

The Health and Safety at Work Act 1974 and the Manual Handling Regulations 1992 give employers responsibilities to assess manual handling tasks, reduce the risk of injury where lifting is unavoidable and to provide equipment such as hoists to enable people to be moved safely. If people are unable to get in and out of the bath with minimal assistance then hoists should be available within the home. It is important that carers use hoists provided for the safety of both the older person and the staff.

Whenever possible the older person should be left alone to bathe in privacy. A call bell should be left within easy reach so that the person can call for help when she has finished bathing. If you are worried that it may be unsafe to leave the person alone to bathe, check with a senior member of staff.

Frail older people may be unable to wash or bath, and staff must carry this out. Registered nurses within the home will show you how this is done. It is important to check if it is safe to leave a frail older person alone in the bathroom, as some may require a carer to remain with them at all times.

Activity 4

 Mrs Doris Frost has just entered the home. Last year she slipped in her bath and broke her wrist trying to save herself. She confesses that she is now terrified of bathing. List ways in which you can help her to remain clean while understanding her fears and respecting her wishes.

COMMENT

It is essential that you listen to Mrs Frost, understand her fears and under no circumstances force her to bathe if she does not wish to do so. You may:

- wish to show her the equipment available to help her get in and out of the bath. Mrs Frost may feel more confident about bathing when she realises that hoists are available and that she will not have to climb in and out of the bath.
- offer to stay with her if she wishes to use the bath, and assure her that you will immediately take her out of the bath if she feels upset.
- show Mrs Frost the showers in the home and offer to help her shower instead of bathing.
- offer to help her to wash at the wash basin and help her to shampoo her hair in the wash basin.

Hair care

In many homes a hairdresser visits once or twice each week to cut, perm and set residents hair. A hairdo is a great morale booster for most women, and carers can help residents to comb and style hair between hairdressing appointments. People who do not have hair shampooed and set by the hairdresser will need their hair washed once or twice per week with a mild shampoo.

Shaving

Many men feel dishevelled and dirty if they are unshaven. Even very disabled men can often manage to shave themselves with an electric razor and a shaving mirror. Carers should encourage individuals to shave themselves whenever possible and offer assistance if required. Senior staff can show you how to shave male patients who are unable to do this for themselves: see Figure 8.4.

Mouth care

Many older people have dentures though some have dental plates and remaining natural teeth. The best way of cleaning both dentures and natural teeth is by using a toothbrush and toothpaste. Whenever possible, individuals should be helped and encouraged to care for their own teeth. When this is not possible, staff must brush the person's teeth. Some people prefer to have their dentures soaked in a soaking solution overnight after cleaning which kills bacteria and prevents mouth infections. Carers should take into account the individual's preference and any policies on mouth care within the home.

Activity 5

Bring your toothbrush and toothpaste from home and arrange for a colleague to do the same. Brush each other's teeth. Discuss how this felt and write down ways in which you can improve the way you brush patients' teeth.

COMMENT

When brushing your colleague's teeth, you probably stood up and loomed over him or her sitting in the chair. This, as you discovered when your teeth were being brushed, can be threatening and frightening. Sitting down on a chair makes the whole procedure less hurried and more friendly. You will also find that approaching the person from the side is more pleasant. Did you remember to offer a mouth wash?

DRESSING

Older people who suffer from a number of medical conditions may find it difficult to dress without help. Carers can advise individuals who are disabled to choose clothes that are easier to take on and off. Suitable clothing can enable older people to regain the ability to dress without help or reduce the amount of help which is required.

- Dresses which fasten at the front are easier to put on.
- Dresses and blouses with wide sleeves are easier to put on than those with tight sleeves.
- Skirts and trousers with elasticated waist bands are easier to put on and more comfortable to wear than those with buttons at the waist band.
- A full skirt is more comfortable to wear than a straight skirt.

People who have difficulty doing up buttons and fasteners may find that:

- Large buttons are easier to fasten.
- Zips are easier to do up than fasteners.
- Elasticated trousers such as jogging pants may be more comfortable than trousers.
- Velcro can be used to fasten clothes together.

Many older people prefer to dress independently. Helping them to choose clothing which is easy to put on and fasten enables many older people to retain independence. Many people find that aids such as the 'helping hand' can help them to put on stockings unaided. If you think that an aid might help an older person, ask a senior member of staff for advice.

Some older people are unable to dress and carers may be required to help or to dress the individual completely. Senior staff within the home will show you how to do this. Remember to give the individual the opportunity to select clothing as you would with a less dependent person.

Activity 6

Mrs Victoria Bruce has just come to live at the home. She recently suffered a stroke and has difficulty dressing. How can you help her to choose clothing which is easy to put on?

COMMENT

1 Suggest that she spends some time practising dressing and finds out which items of clothing in her wardrobe are easiest to put on and take off.
2 Suggest that her family adapt some of her other clothing so that she can dress more easily.
3 Ask a senior member of staff to show Mrs Bruce special methods of dressing which take account of her disability.
4 Encourage Mrs Bruce to persevere, but be ready to offer help if needed.

INCONTINENCE

Maintaining continence

Older people can develop incontinence of the bladder or bowel. This can be very distressing for the older person and the carer. Both may feel that incontinence is due to old age and that little can be done to help.

However, incontinence is a symptom of illness, and many factors can lead to an older person developing it. A bladder infection, the effects of medication and treatable medical conditions can all lead to this symptom. It is important that carers are aware that in many cases incontinence can be successfully treated. If an older person becomes incontinent, this should be reported to a senior member of staff who will arrange for it to be investigated and treated.

Older people who retain the ability to use the toilet without help are less likely to develop continence problems. People who are not rushed and who are treated with dignity, respect and privacy will feel less anxious. Anxiety, unhappiness and depression can make people more likely to become incontinent. Older people living in homes may require help to walk to the toilet and are less able to wait than younger people.

- It is important that carers respond quickly to requests to help a person to the toilet. The older person may be unable to hold on while you finish laying the tables.

CASE HISTORY 8

Mr George Jenkins has lived at Ambleside residential home for some time. Recently he suffered from a bleeding ulcer and was admitted to hospital. When he returned to the home he had lost control of his bowels and bladder. Staff reported this to his General Practitioner (GP) who asked the continence adviser to see Mr Jenkins, to find out why he had become incontinent.

The continence adviser discovered that Mr Jenkins had been prescribed iron tablets. These had caused severe constipation. The constipation had led to fluid leaking from the bowel and staff had mistaken this for diarrhoea. The mass of constipated faeces had caused urinary incontinence.

Treating the constipation and offering high fibre foods and plenty of fluids enabled Mr Jenkins to regain bowel and bladder control.

Caring for individuals who suffer from incontinence

Some individuals who suffer from incontinence cannot be helped to regain control of

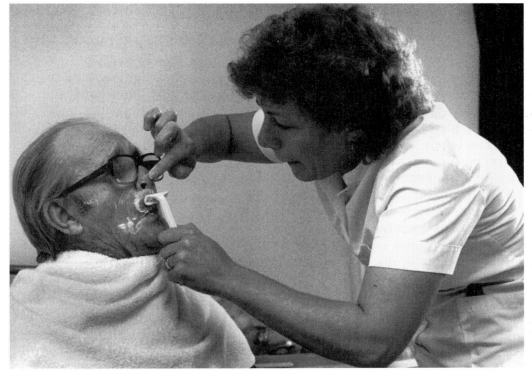

Figure 8.4   Shaving a client is a delicate duty

the bladder or bowels. In such cases the aims of care are:

- to contain incontinence
- to ensure that the person is treated with dignity and respect
- to prevent complications such as sore skin from developing.

Information on the methods used to achieve these aims will be recorded in the care plan and senior staff at the home can advise you.

Activity 7

 Consider ways in which you help people in the home remain continent.

COMMENT

 Your list should include the following:

1 Make sure that patients are always able to reach the call bell, and can call for assistance.
2 If the person is able to walk to the toilet using a frame, make sure this is always within reach.
3 Respond promptly when asked to assist a person to the toilet.
4 Help the person maintain dignity and privacy by making sure that toilet doors are closed and bed curtains are pulled when the toilet or commode is being used.
5 If the person is incontinent, inform a senior member of staff so that the reasons for this can be investigated and treatment offered.

PRESSURE SORES

Pressure sores are often known as bedsores, although a person does not have to be confined to bed to develop one. They are caused by pressure or friction on an area of the body, which cuts off the supply of blood to the tissues and causes a pressure sore to develop.

Most pressure sores can be prevented. People who are unable to move can develop pressure sores on any part of the body. The most common places are on the sacrum, buttocks, hips and heels. Encouraging and helping older people to move around helps prevent pressure sores developing.

People living in nursing homes are usually more frail and more at risk of developing pressure sores than those living in residential homes. Registered nurses in nursing homes assess the individual's risk of developing pressure sores and work out a plan of care to prevent their development. The treatment usually includes using special mattress overlays, mattresses and special cushions, and changing the person's position frequently.

Activity 8

 Ask a senior member of staff in the home you are visiting or working in, to identify a person in the home who is at risk of developing pressure sores. Identify and list the reasons why the person is at risk. Note the care which is given to prevent pressure sores developing, and the equipment used to reduce pressure.

COMMENT

1 The person whom you have identified will be unable to move around in bed or in a chair.
2 The person may be underweight or overweight. Underweight people are at risk because their bones are more prominent, which will encourage pressure sores. Overweight people are at risk because fat has a poorer blood supply than lean tissue.
3 The person may be confused. Confused

people are at greater risk because they may be unaware that they have been sitting or lying in one position for a long time, and that their skin is becoming sore.
4 The person might be a diabetic. Some people with diabetes have reduced sensation to the skin and may not realise that they are becoming sore.

CARE

All nursing care aims to relieve pressure on the body. People who are sitting may be helped to stand up or walk. People who are in bed may be helped to turn over.

EQUIPMENT

Nurses will use a range of equipment designed to spread the person's weight over a large area and reduce the effects of pressure:

- Elbow and heel protectors are used to prevent pressure sores developing on these areas.
- A range of cushions will be used within the home to suit the needs of individuals.
- A range of mattress overlays and mattress replacement systems, from foam overlays to alternating pressure overlays and mattresses, will be used according to the degree of risk each individual faces.

HELPING OLDER PEOPLE TO EAT

Many older people have difficulty eating because of the effects of illness or disability. Some have difficulty holding cutlery, others may find food slips off the plate or that the plate slips on the table. People who have poor vision may be unable to see light coloured food on a white plate.

- Using aids such as special easy-to-grip cutlery, plate guards which prevent food sliding off a plate, non-slip mats to prevent food slipping and dark coloured plates to enable people to see the food, can enable people to feed themselves.

- People who have dentures which no longer fit will have difficulty in eating. A dental surgeon can alter dentures so that they are more comfortable or make new dentures.
- Most people prefer to feed themselves rather than to be fed. A few people will require feeding. If feeding a person, the carer should always sit down to the side of the person and take time to ensure the person enjoys the meal, is not rushed, and is offered drinks throughout the meal. Senior staff in your home will be able to offer further guidance and help.

COMMUNICATING WITH OLDER PEOPLE

Carers may find it difficult to communicate with some individuals because they have problems with hearing or speech. Over 7.5 million people in UK have hearing loss. Hearing deteriorates as people get older: 60 per cent of 70-year-olds and 90 per cent of 90-year-olds suffer from hearing loss. This affects the ability to understand and respond to carers and to others living in the home.

Unfortunately, people with poor hearing may be thought to be confused or may get left out of conversations. Others are inclined to think that deaf people are not 'with it'. Many older people with hearing loss find communicating with others extremely frustrating, and if they feel that people are ignoring them, talking over them or treating them as though they were senile, they may simply give up trying to communicate. As one lady with hearing loss stated 'If they make no effort, why should I bother?'. Carers who make an effort to communicate with older people with hearing loss can encourage them to communicate with other people, and take part in the daily life of the home.

Hearing aids

People who have difficulty hearing are normally sent to see the Ear, Nose and Throat specialist at the local hospital. Hearing is tested in the out-patient's clinic, where the type and causes of deafness are identified. In many cases a hearing aid is supplied.

ENCOURAGING OLDER PEOPLE TO USE THEIR HEARING AIDS

Many older people do not use their hearing aids. In one survey of homes, half of the older people who had hearing aids did not wear them. The reasons the older people gave were that they found them difficult to put in and adjust, or that the aids no longer worked. To ensure correct use of a hearing aid:

1 Ear pieces must be fitted firmly into the ear if the aid is to work.
2 Aids must be turned on, and turned to the correct setting. The setting varies from individual to individual, but should be set at the level which enables the older person to hear easily.
3 Batteries must be changed regularly.

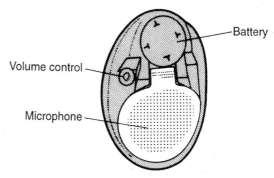

Figure 8.5   A hearing aid

These simple tasks take only a few minutes but enable older people to communicate with carers. This saves time and reduces frustration throughout the day.

Hearing aids do not restore hearing to normal: they work by amplifying all sound, including background noises. Carers can make it easier for people with hearing aids to hear by following these points:

- Reduce background noise. Close the door and window if it is noisy outside.
- Face the person, move near and face the light.
- Speak a little more loudly than usual, but don't shout. Shouting distorts the voice making it more difficult to hear, and appears threatening.
- Speak directly to the person. Do not attempt to have conversations with more than one person at the same time. The deaf person will have difficulty following this.
- Do not cover your mouth while speaking.
- Speak slowly and clearly.
- If you have not been understood, use different words with similar meanings.
- Check that the individual has understood.
- Use gestures.
- Offer to write things down.

Activity 9

 Identify some of the reasons that older people may have difficulty communicating.

COMMENT

 Your list should include:

1 People who are deaf.
2 People who have difficulty speaking.
3 People who have difficulty understanding what you say.

4 People who have had strokes or who suffer from diseases such as Parkinsons's disease may have difficulty pronouncing words.
5 Some people who have had strokes may have difficulty understanding what we say – our words no longer make sense to them.
6 People who are suffering from dementia may have difficulty understanding us because their concentration is poor, understanding is limited and we are too rushed.

Activity 10

 Outline ways in which you can help people who have difficulties in communicating to make themselves understood.

COMMENT

 Your list should include:

1 Spend time with the person, get to know him or her, gain her confidence. The person will be more relaxed and find communicating easier.
2 Do not appear busy and rushed (even if you are), as this will make the person anxious and make communication more difficult.
3 Sit down.
4 Face the person.
5 Use short sentences.
6 Speak slowly and clearly.
7 Listen to what the person is saying.
8 Check that you have understood.

MAINTAINING SELF ESTEEM WITHIN A HOME

Older people who enter homes understandably feel anxious. It is important that older people are treated as individuals and that they are listened to.

- The person should be addressed by their preferred title; this may be Mrs Stevens, Maude, or even a nickname.
- The home should have policies which ensure that the person is treated sensitively and with respect.
- Visitors should be welcomed and the individual encouraged to maintain activities and interests which were pursued at home. It is normally possible for the individual to continue to attend church services or other activities which he or she took part in at home.
- Most homes have activities programmes and carers are involved in these.
- Staff should treat the older person with respect: knocking before entering their room, finding out what their preferences are and working with them in partnership to offer care which is tailored to their individual needs.

SUMMARY

People living in homes come from a variety of backgrounds and have a wide range of abilities. They are cared for in different care settings, because they require different levels of care. In all care settings and regardless of the level of their disabilities, people should be offered care which is based on their needs and preferences. Care is provided by Registered nurses and care assistants working together with older people to provide care of the highest quality.

Further information

These charities offer further information:

The Arthritis & Rheumatism Council for Research (ARC)
Copeman House,
St Mary's Court,
Chesterfield,
Derbyshire, S41 7TD
Telephone: 01246 558033

ARC is a charity which provides information for patients, carers, doctors and nurses. They produce a wide range of leaflets and booklets. Single copies are available free of charge. ARC will provide full details of their publications on request.

The Stroke Association
CHSA House,
Whitecross Street,
London, EC1 8JJ.
Telephone: 0171 490 2686

The Stroke Association provide telephone help-lines; support to over 400 stroke clubs, fund research into the causes of stroke and offer information about how to reduce the risk of stroke. They produce free leaflets including information on physiotherapy and occupational therapy. They also produce books and videos.

The British Association of the Hard of Hearing (Hearing Concern)
7–11, Armstrong Road,
London, W3 7JL
Telephone: 0181 743 1110

The Sympathetic Hearing Scheme aims to make people more aware of hearing difficulties. It produces leaflets and educational material. It has a network of volunteers and may be able to provide a volunteer speaker to visit the nursing or residential home where you work or your college. They also produce an excellent video which can be hired.

Further reading

All the books mentioned are suitable for care assistants. You may be able to obtain them from your college library.

Jenkins, J. (1992), The clothes in question. Scutari Press, Harrow.

This book gives advice and information on choosing, adapting and caring for patient's clothes when they are living in homes.

Disabled Living Foundation (1994) All dressed up. Disabled Living Foundation, London.

This book is full of practical advice and tips on choosing and adapting clothes. It also provides elderly people with advice on how to dress. There is a section on how to dress people who are unable to dress themselves.

Fader, M., Norton, C., (1994), Caring for continence. Hawker Publications Ltd, London.

This book has been written specially for care assistants studying at NVQ level two and three. It costs £4.50 + 75p post and packaging and is available from: Hawker Publications Ltd, 13 Park House, 140, Battersea Park Road, London SW11 4NB.

Castledean, Prof C. M., Duffin, H. (1988), Staying Dry. Advice for sufferers of incontinence. Quay Publishing, 11 Victoria Wharf, St George's Quay, Lancaster, LA1 1GA.

This book is aimed at people who suffer from incontinence. It is simple and easy to understand and carers will find it useful. It is available in large bookshops.

Norton, C. (1986), Nursing for Continence. Beaconsfield Publishers Ltd, 20 Chiltern Hills Road, Beaconsfield, Buckinghamshire, HP9 1PL.

This book although written for the trained nurse is easy to read and a full explanation of all terms used is given. It will interest carers who require more detailed information.

Benson, S. (ed.) (1995), Care Assistants Handbooks. A series of handbooks for care assistants working with different client groups in care settings. Hawker Publications, 13 Park House, 140 Battersea Park Road, London SW1 4NB.

Nazarko, L. (1996), NVQs in Nursing & Residential Homes. Blackwell Scientific, Oxford. Covers the work of care assistants within care homes in greater detail.

Telephone helplines

A number of organisations have a telephone service. Carers can telephone and ask for advice and information.

- The Bard Helpline is open from 12.30–4.30 pm Monday to Friday. Telephone 0800 591 783
- Coloplast Service help line is open from 9.00 am until 7.00 pm Monday to Friday. Telephone 0800 220 622
- Hollister Incare Helpline is open from 9.00 am until 5.00 pm Monday to Friday. Telephone 0800 521 377
- The Incontinence Information Helpline is run by a charity and offers advice and help. The lines are open from 9.00 a.m. until 7.00 pm Monday to Friday. Telephone 0191 213 0050.

INDEX